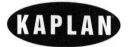

Other Kaplan Books Related to Nursing and Professional Development

NCLEX-RN with CD-ROM

Going Indie: Self-Employment, Freelance, & Temping Opportunities

Résumé Builder & Career Counselor

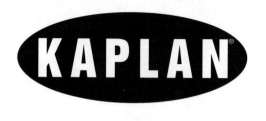

Careers in Nursing

Managing Your Future in the Changing World of Healthcare

By Annette Vallano, M.S., R.N., C.S., N.P.

Simon & Schuster

Kaplan Books

Published by Kaplan Educational Centers and Simon & Schuster
1230 Avenue of the Americas
New York, NY 10020

Project Editor: Richard Christiano
Cover Design: Cheung Tai
Interior Illustrations: Jude Bond
Production Editor: Maude Spekes
Desktop Publishing Manager: Michael Shevlin
Managing Editor: David Chipps
Executive Editor: Del Franz

Special thanks are extended to Eileen Mager, Jin Jie Li, Judi Knott, and Linda Volpano.

Manufactured in the United States of America. Published simultaneously in Canada.

February 1999
10 9 8 7 6 5 4 3

Library of Congress Cataloging-in-Publication Data is available.

ISBN: 0-684-85236-5

Table of Contents

Many Books Offer Career Advice for Nurses. What Makes This Book Different?

This book explains how to treat your career as if it were an entrepreneur's venture—a necessity in today's changing healthcare industry. No other book blends the lessons learned in business with your own values and career so well. The sweeping changes brought about by managed care do *not* mean that nurses can no longer enjoy career security. In fact, you can enjoy an even greater sense of confidence and independence by reading and acting on the advice in *Careers in Nursing.* Some books contain only on-the-job advice, while others rely too heavily on inspirational—but nonpractical—essays.

Careers in Nursing **is designed to help you improve both your career *and* your life** by focusing on matching your values and needs to the job you have ... or the job you want. Whatever your nursing obstacle is—hospital downsizing, outdated skills, writing a résumé, or just common, everyday stress—this book will show you how to get your career back on track.

About the Author

Annette Vallano is a clinical nurse specialist and nurse practitioner in psychiatric mental health nursing in private practice in New York City. She is founder and director of The Self Care Center for Nurses, established in 1987 to teach and promote self care and personal empowerment strategies for nurses. Annette is an adjunct member of the nursing faculties of Mercy College in Dobbs Ferry, New York, and New York University, and is currently the mental health clinician for Lenox Hill Hospital's home care department. Annette also serves as a consultant to healthcare organizations, such as the New York Hospital–Cornell Medical Center.

Annette has already transformed her nursing career several times. A diploma graduate of St. John's Episcopal Hospital in Brooklyn, New York, she received her B.S.N. and M.S. from Adelphi University. She has been a staff nurse and a nurse manager, working in pediatric, obstetrical, and psychiatric nursing after serving in the U.S. Army Nurse Corps. Her extensive nursing experience gives her firsthand knowledge of the complexities, joys, challenges, and rewards of nursing practice, and she is committed to preserving and enhancing the personal and professional well-being of nurses.

Dedication

To the enduring and supportive memory of Evelyn Zalewski, M.A., R.N.,
nurse, teacher, mentor, healer, with eternal gratitude and affection.

PART ONE

The New Frontier
of Healthcare

Chapter 1

The Healthcare Revolution

The Best of Times or the Worst of Times?

At the turn of the century we stand before a new dawn in healthcare and a new frontier for nurses. Just as the American Revolution shaped the United States we live in today, so the Healthcare Revolution is shaping the future of healthcare delivery systems as well as nursing practice. As the entire world of work, including the healthcare workplace, is being transformed, so must we, as nurses, transform our relationship to this new world, and perhaps with ourselves as well. Whether these are the best of times or the worst of times depends on your perspective and your ability to manage change. It will seem more like the best of times if you are riding the horse in the direction it's going, rather than facing backwards, trying to recreate the past.

> "Our deepest fear is not that we are inadequate. Our deepest fear is that we are powerful beyond measure. It is our light, not our darkness, that most frightens us. We ask ouselves, who am I to be brilliant, gorgeous, talented, and fabulous? Actually, who are you not to be? You are a child of God. Your playing small doesn't serve the world. . . . As we are liberated from our own fear, our presence automatically liberates others."
>
> —Nelson Mandela, from his 1994 inaugural speech

You can experience these changes as the best of times if you learn to be a proactive explorer and trend watcher, living along the outer edges of your comfort zone as you reach ever forward, aligning yourself with the new opportunities change always creates. By developing strategies to meet the challenge of change and reframe situations to see the optimistic and opportunistic sides of them, you will not only survive, but thrive professionally and personally.

Nurses who feel defeated by change, who resist learning the new workplace rules, who believe they are powerless victims without choice or control, who use rumor rather than fact as a source of information—they will be infected with doom and gloom and will be convinced that these are the worst of times. These nurses are in danger of being tossed about by the winds of change. A newspaper ad of the early 1990s captured the essence of this idea well:

Change is
inevitable.
Those who cannot
manage change
successfully
will
vanish

To align most effectively with this new world of work, you need to learn how to use the Healthcare Revolution as a spark for your own evolution, as a way to ignite new levels of professional and personal growth. New skills, new attitudes and values, and new ways of working and thinking about work will evolve with your motivation to change, seek support when necessary, and obtain accurate information. This is what can make it the best of times for you.

For some nurses, the Healthcare Revolution may evoke a professional or a personal crisis, especially if they are unprepared—like the nurse caught by surprise by a redesigned role or a downsized position. In the Chinese language the meaning of the word *crisis* is embedded in its symbol for *opportunity*, which is translated to mean both trouble and crisis.

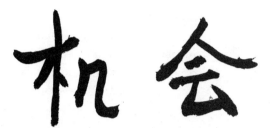

Trouble + Crisis = Opportunity

In psychological terms, a crisis can occur when there is a disruption in the homeostatic balance, the status quo of one's life, resulting in the paradox of danger and opportunity existing together. When a change, expected or unexpected, is perceived as a challenge rather than a threat, the potential crisis can generally be averted. Accurate perception, adequate support, and effective coping are three balancing factors that not only influence whether or not a crisis occurs, but also its three potential outcomes of thriving and growth, survival and stagnation, or collapse and regression. Nurses who are thriving and growing as a result of the Healthcare Revolution are those who work toward:

- Accurately perceiving the meaning and impact of the changes
- Establishing networks for support and information
- Learning to live and cope in an era of constant change and permanent transition

Of course, nurses who thrive are not immune from being bewildered, exasperated, and stressed by these changes. What makes them thrivers, however, is that rather than being victimized and defeated by change, they reach for the opportunities in it and are challenged by the adventure of it. You may, at times, pessimistically perceive the glass as half empty. What you must strengthen, however, is your capacity to also recognize the half-filled nature of the glass, and how to shift to what can encourage, rather than defeat you, namely what is in the glass, rather than what is not.

Another way to envision these three outcomes is to imagine yourself in a boat with other people, rowing down a river, when suddenly the water becomes turbulent as it moves through smaller spaces and drops onto the uneven surfaces of half-hidden rocks. This condition, known as whitewater, is actually sought out in the sport of whitewater rafting. *Permanent whitewater* is a term used by Jane Schuman in her article,

> "Man can learn nothing except going from the known to the unknown."
>
> —Claude Bernard

"Navigating the Whitewater of Change" (*American Journal of Nursing*), as a metaphor to describe the permanent condition of continuous, accelerated change occurring in organizations today. Schuman goes on to describe three typical responses to the crisis of finding yourself in permanent whitewater. The responses closely match the outcomes of a crisis situation as described above. Reflect on each of the descriptions below and ask yourself which might best describe your response?

The Victim: You expect the worst and are sure that danger is just around the next bend. You are reactive rather than proactive and spend a lot of time gripping the side of the raft with white-knuckled terror, blaming and criticizing those trying to steer.

The Survivor: You have your life jacket buckled securely and will stay afloat, but believe you are only along for the ride and therefore have no choice about the direction of the boat and no power to influence anything in the situation.

The Navigator: You see your changing situation as an adventure. You are scared at times, but get through the swelling currents by developing new rafting skills or strengthening the old ones. Your confidence grows in proportion to your ability to work with those who are doing the steering.

The ability to become change-hardy by developing and strengthening stress management strategies is what can influence you to be a navigator rather than a survivor or a victim. It is not so much the intensity of the change that determines which of these three outcomes will occur, but the degree of control you believe you have over your destiny. Your ability to navigate through permanent whitewater while also controlling the direction of your nursing practice relies on strengthening related skills and strategies while managing the stress that may accompany it all. Think of your nursing life as supported by a three-legged stool: One leg is your clinical and professional competencies, another leg stands for your career development skills and strategies, and the third leg your stress management strategies (or self care). A stool requires its legs to be equal in length to remain stable. So these three "legs" of your nursing life need equal shaping and attention. Neglect one for too long a period of time, and the imbalance could knock you off track.

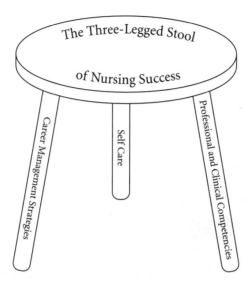

The Three-Legged Stool

of Nursing Success

Career Management Strategies

Self Care

Professional and Clinical Competencies

The following stories describe three nurses who are facing the same dilemma with varying degrees of success. As you read about Nancy, Vera, and Cora, decide which nurse most closely resembles you.

Profile of a Navigator: Nancy

A member of her medical center's IV Team for five years, Nancy was not caught off guard when her role was redesigned. She saw the handwriting on the wall when the medical center merged with another hospital whose direct care nurses started their own IVs, rather than relying on a centralized team. She decided not to accept the offer of being reassigned to an inpatient unit because she relishes the freedom she's now enjoying. She likes moving around from unit to unit, planning her own schedule, and responding with autonomy to patient needs. She wants to utilize the high-tech IV skills she's honed so carefully, even though she felt confused and worried initially about where and how to do this. At a career strategy seminar she learned about sign-on bonuses in home care for nurses with her skills, so she decided to make the move. The adaptation to a new kind of nursing environment was rocky at first but is now quite smooth. She even finds herself smiling as she walks down the street, carrying nursing supplies in her backpack while traveling between patients' homes, wondering why she hadn't done this sooner. Not only does she have more freedom and autonomy than before, she has sunshine and exercise too!

Profile of a Survivor: Vera

Vera feels blown into the water by the force of change and is using all her energy to hold on to her job as if it were a life raft, not recognizing that her job is different from her career. She is unable to navigate into new professional or personal waters. She desperately looks for another position as an IV nurse, only to discover that most other organizations have also shifted this role to the direct care nurse or will soon do so. She considers herself fortunate when she is one of two nurses from the IV Team who are retained to act as educational resources to nurses needing extra assistance as they learn to start their own IVs. When Vera is advised that this position is only temporary, she makes statements like, "Maybe they'll change their mind. They'll see how indispensable this role is and decide to keep me." She is in danger of being lulled into the same rhythm of familiar repetition that resulted in her shock at being downsized to begin with. The comfort of this routine may numb her alertness to the signals around her. Vera has survived, but is vulnerable to a cycle of stagnant repetition that is potentially stressful as well as self-defeating. She is looking backward, trying to recreate the past rather than see the opportunities ahead.

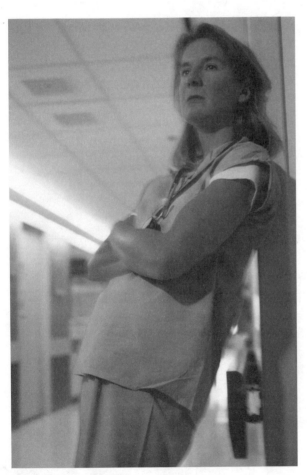

How do you deal with nursing stress? Are you a navigator, a survivor, or a victim?

Profile of a Victim: Cora

Cora feels too lost to see or move into what's next for her. She feels defeated and perceives being downsized as a betrayal, and is unable to alter her view. She feels forced into retiring early, even though she does not feel ready. She wonders if she should look for work elsewhere in nursing or even leave healthcare completely. She is considering what it would be like to live on only her spouse's income. Cora finds herself withdrawn and depressed, unable to shake the bronchitis that developed following the cold she had last winter. Some people might confuse Cora's response with that of a nurse who takes advantage of the time after being downsized to create a self-designed sabbatical. The responses are not the same, however: The nurse on sabbatical is proactively taking control of her destiny, while Cora is allowing her control to slip away.

The important lesson for you is not so much whether your experience is like Cora's or Vera's, but whether you know how to turn it into something closer to Nancy's. Or at least believe that you can! That's the power of the "half-filled glass" metaphor. Your capacity to find optimism and allow it to influence and generate positive feelings is a potent self-care strategy—a leg of your three-legged stool that should not be underestimated.

The People in the Parentheses

We have become what psychologist and human-potential expert Jean Houston calls "the people in the parentheses": those people suspended between what was and what will be as the healthcare system performs its dismantling and restructuring dance. We belong to the generation of nurses bridging the gap between old and new, past and future, now and to be. Life within the parentheses is both challenging and threatening to our professional and personal wholeness, integrity, and well-being as we struggle to maintain our footing in a constantly changing work environment.

John Naisbett, author of *Megatrends: Ten New Directions for Transforming Our Lives*, echoes this by saying:

> We are living in the time of the parentheses, the time between eras. Those who are willing to handle the ambiguity of this in-between period and to anticipate the new era will be a quantum leap ahead of those who hold on to the past. The time of the parentheses is a time of change and questioning. Although the time between eras is uncertain, it is a great and yeasty time, filled with opportunity. If we can learn to make uncertainty our friend, we can achieve much more than in stable eras. In stable eras, every-

thing has a name, and everything knows its place and we can leverage very little. But in the time of the parenthesis we have extraordinary leverage and influence, individually, professionally, and institutionally, if we can get a clear sense, a clear conception, a clear vision, of the road ahead. My God, what a fantastic time to be alive!"

People in the parentheses can feel off track in their lives. Being temporarily off track is sometimes necessary because it can signal the need to move from where you've been to where you need to go. It is common to find yourself in a disorienting place during this Healthcare Revolution; where your values and vision may no longer match those of your old workplace, where what has worked before no longer does. In this place you may be questioning what you are doing and why it matters. You may feel bored and out of touch with what you like about nursing. You may call this experience burnout if the work you were once committed to now creates more mental confusion and emotional fatigue than before. You may mistakenly blame the people in the organization you work for rather than decide whether you still want to be on the same track as they are or find a new track more aligned with your mission, values, and vision. You will have opportunities to explore this in chapter 7, "Product Development."

Being off track signals that you may be ready for new professional challenges. This is not necessarily a new experience for nurses who have long benefited from this flexibility of options and opportunities inherent in the nursing career path. What is different today is that the time to make a career shift is more often dictated by changes in the workplace than controlled by you.

For example, many nurses working in acute care hospitals are finding their careers off track as these hospitals shift to caring for sicker patients who stay for shorter lengths of time despite the acuity of their illness. These patients require more high-tech care, utilizing complex life-sustaining technology. This new work environment may no longer support the lengthier patient contact valued by the nurse. Shorter lengths of stay mean shortened relationships with patients in which teaching, emotional support, and discharge planning must be accomplished in less time. Nurses who value these nursing competencies may find themselves off track without them.

So being off track is an important and essential signal for all nurses, including acute-care nurses, to plot a new career path to a nursing practice environment that would more closely match their nursing skills and competencies, mission, values, as well as their vision. Likewise, they may decide to adapt to the changes that are occurring and learn the skills and competencies now associated with acute care hospitals.

Each of these scenarios is currently being played out by nurses at California's Kaiser Permanente Hospital, the nation's biggest health maintenance organization, where the role of Accelerated-Care Nurse has been introduced. As reported in the New York Times (April 9, 1998) by Peter T. Kilborn, one nurse "snapped her fingers in describing the speed with which she and the nurses she supervises in the new 21-bed Short-Stay Unit perform their tasks . . . as they move patients from suture to discharge in under 48 hours." As described in the article, a nurse with 16 years of experience has mixed feelings now that the essence of the work she loves—the nurturing in nursing—is vanishing. She goes on to say, "My passion was getting to know my patients, their identity, their hearts, their souls. I would rather know a few patients well than fragments of many."

Another nurse felt quite differently about this accelerated role as she described the reduced fragmentation of

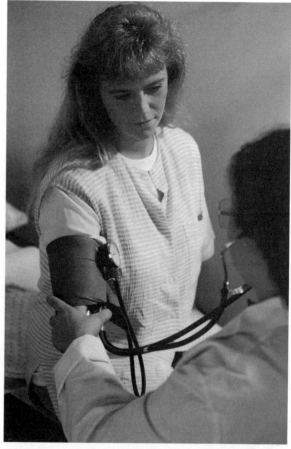

The new acute-care workplace, where shorter stays are the rule, may no longer support the lengthier contact valued by the nurse.

patient care achieved by doing what once took at least two other healthcare workers to do: "In the short-stay unit now, I draw the blood, do the EKG, and teach patients about medications. It's faster when you can do it all. For me, it's more fulfilling."

You may be experiencing something similar to this, or perhaps you're concerned that you soon will. Cora, Nancy, and Vera were temporarily off track and used different strategies to get back on. Which might be more useful to your situation, adapting or moving on? Which of these nurses' experiences do you think might best describe you?

What's important here is not so much which option you choose to get back on track, but that you make a conscious choice based on your needs, how you want to practice nursing, and what is best for you in response to these workplace shifts. What is essential is that you update and clarify your vision, your mission, and your values, just as the organization you work for is updating and clarifying theirs. These three essential components of your nursing practice are tools that can clarify which track you should be on as the world of work changes. They will also help you to discover how much control you really do have, and where along the Continuum of Care (the process by which the patient will receive healthcare services along a pathway that spans the gamut between wellness and prevention of illness on one end, to rehabilitation or long term care on the other end) your work skills and nursing competencies would be best utilized. This book will help you identify your vision, your mission, and your values and use them to keep your career on track.

The next chapter, "What's Changing and Why," will be your first step towards embracing change by providing an introduction to the changes the Healthcare Revolution is bringing about.

Chapter 2

What's Changing and Why

The Healthcare Revolution began when broad-reaching social, political, and economic factors united to create unprecedented changes in the workplace of all North American industries. The introduction by Medicare of prospective payment for preidentified, diagnostic-related groups in the 1980s, was the precursor of the managed-care systems of the 1990s. This has led to the need for predicting and controlling the patients' length of stay, and to the development of clinical pathways that ensure compliance with standards and control of expensive resources. The government and employers, who once paid almost blindly for healthcare costs, have become more like watchdogs than passive payers. This new intrusion in the management of patient care has rocked the healthcare industry. The changes of the 1980s turned out to be a small tremor compared to the earthquake occurring as the new millennium begins.

> "The two things I hear most are that things will stay exactly the way they are and that things will change."
>
> —Brad Lampert

Today, led by organizational consultants, healthcare is forced to apply business practices to its disorganized and cost-overrun systems. It must not only reinvent how it manages its care, but also how it organizes and provides its services while determining how to finance them. Hence the appearance of managed care systems, as well as terms like *restructuring*, *reengineering*, and *redesigning*, all entering the vocabulary and shaking the psyche of every healthcare worker. This new terminology can destroy your long-held sense of security—both personally and professionally.

> "The jolting changes we are experiencing are not chaotic or random but, in fact, they form a sharp, clearly discernible pattern . . . . Moreover, these changes are cumulative—they add up to a giant transformation in the way we live, work, play, and think."
>
> —Alvin Toffler, *The Third Wave*

The management of healthcare organizations is being restructured, leading to a more efficient and less costly flattening of administrative hierarchies with fewer middle managers. Head nurses, for example, are now known as nurse managers, reflecting the emerging scope of their responsibilities. A shortened pecking order between the executive in charge of the organization and the nurse at the bedside is emerging. Directors of nursing are more likely to be called vice presidents as their responsibilities and influence widen. Patient care processes such as admission and discharge procedures are being reengineered to be more efficient, more economical, and more user-friendly. Also, the ways in which the actual work of patient care gets done—who is doing what, where, and for how long—is being redesigned.

While all three of these processes—reengineering, restructuring, and redesign—directly influence your role as a nurse, the one that probably has the most direct impact is the redesign of the nursing role using unlicensed assistive personnel. These workers, sometimes called *patient care technicians*, were hired to further streamline patient care services. Some see this as an attempt to replace the more costly professional nurse with a less costly, nonprofessional technician. While the practical reasons for creating this kind of role include relieving you of some technical, non-nursing functions, it is also seen as an attempt by some organizations to cut their costs in ways that often wind up delivering a lower standard of nursing care. This has resulted in the creation of two conflicts for you as a nurse. The first has to do with the loss of your role, perhaps even your job. The second has to do with what, as a patient advocate, you should do about the lower standard of care you often perceive as a result.

While it is true that some hospitals have taken the low road to cost-cutting by dangerously reducing the number of RN jobs, this is not true across the board. In fact, this reduction may be an essential and quite possibly useful stage along the way to changing the workplace mix of the healthcare team. It may actually increase efficiency, productivity, and marketplace competition, and may end up making the best use of your professional talents. Among other things, work redesign attempts to address the longtime professional nursing dilemma of spending too much time performing non-nursing functions. However, like any new change, more time and experience is needed to determine how best to use the patient care technician to this end. For now, it is left to individual nurses and their professional voice, the American Nurses Association, to speak up against this potentially dangerous practice.

As acute care hospitals shift to a "sicker and quicker" mode of care, patient care is extending itself to less costly postacute care locations, such as transitional hospitals, subacute care centers, and home care services. This enriched Continuum of Care has created a wealth of work options and opportunities for nurses that will be explored in chapter 8, "Marketplace Research."

The Essential Truths about the Changing World of Work

There are some essential truths about the changing world of work—and the health-care industry in particular—that should reassure any of you who fear the demise of your profession or erroneously believe you can never recover from the loss of your job security.

Healthcare is a Growth Industry

It is hard to find a list of hot-track careers that doesn't have healthcare on it some-where. Two of the fastest growing segments of healthcare are psychiatric home care and high-tech home care, the result of the expanding Continuum of Care into post-acute and community-based services. Additionally, there are specific segments of the industry that are experiencing such rapid growth that some areas of the country are offering sign-on bonuses! These often include inpatient or community-based high-tech and critical care work.

Healthcare Needs Are Predicted to Increase

Only jobs are being downsized, not accidents, illnesses, births, or deaths! Healthcare needs are predicted to increase, as a result of many social factors, not the least of which is the aging of one of the largest segments of our population: the Baby Boomers.

There Is Still a Nursing Shortage

Despite the difficulty nurses have had locating jobs in the 1990s, there is still a nursing shortage! Paradoxes like this are common during these times of change. The truth is that an increased need for professional nurses has been a constant throughout the 1990s despite a purposeful reduction in the RN workforce as hospitals scramble to cut costs. This is supported by the United States Bureau of Labor Statistics, which predicts an increased need for nurses between the years 1990 to 2020. *The Seventh Report to Congress: Status of Health Care Personnel in the United States* projected this dramatic shift in the availability and need for nursing personnel, with the greatest need for the baccalaureate-prepared nurse. According to their report, more than one million BSN nurses will be needed but less than 600,000 will be available.

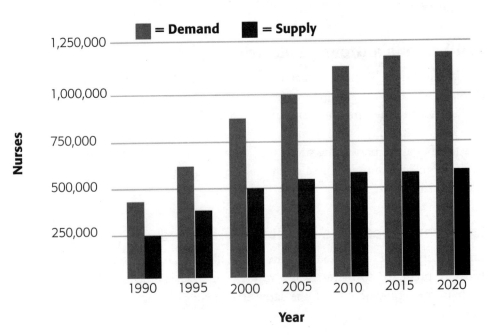

Source: The College Network

Put all these truths together and you have the most reassuring truth of all: There is career security for you if you learn how to play the workplace game by its new rules, including increased self-reliance and interdependence, the willingness to take risks, and the flexibility to adapt to rapid change.

Security doesn't come from a job. It comes from within. It comes from an inner knowing that you can take care of yourself and rely on yourself, no matter what the challenge! Helen Keller might have said it best in the following three quotes:

> "Life is either a daring adventure or nothing."

> "Security is mostly superstition. It does not exist in nature . . . . Avoiding danger is no safer in the long run than outright exposure."

> "To keep our faces towards change and behave like free spirits in the presence of fate is strength undefeatable."

Today a new stage in the Healthcare Revolution is emerging. The nursing surplus is beginning to look more like a nursing shortage again in some areas of the country and in some nursing specialties such as high-tech home care and critical care. This does not mean that employment opportunities and practices will be what they were prior to the Healthcare Revolution. Rather, it signals that a new stage in the revolution is occurring. A revolution means just that: a revolt that permanently shakes up the status quo. There is no going back. The healthcare system is evolving into a different place, for both the patient/consumer and for you.

The "guaranteed" job security experienced by previous generations of nurses will not return. What will replace it is lifelong career security in a growth industry with ever-increasing work options and opportunities for you if you are willing to be proactive, self-reliant, and self-motivated. What you will need for career mobility and employability these days is a willingness to take more responsibility for shaping your career. You can no longer passively rely on a single employer to guarantee work in exchange for your loyalty. Expecting to be "taken care of" in the form of employment benefits or automatic salary increases in exchange for years of "loyal" service transforms what should be a business arrangement between an employer and employee into a kind of dysfunctional dependence. This can slowly erode your freedom and self-reliance, as well as narrow your vision of possibilities. Leah Curtin, the editor of *Nursing Management*, described this well in a 1995 editorial:

Nurses must learn to redirect their loyalty from their employer to their work, committing themselves to self development and skills enlargement. As they invest in themselves, they become more valuable.

If you want to work and move around effectively in this newly recreated system, you must loosen the bonds of organizational dependence and learn how to play the new game with its new rules to follow and new challenges to meet. Some of these challenges relate to your clinical and professional skills, others are about self-care and stress management, and still others concern the development of proactive and assertive career strategies. This trio of skills creates the three-legged stool mentioned in the previous chapter, with each leg needing to be of equal length and strength to achieve career success. The stool must stand firm in order to act as the antidote to stress and burnout.

Is Healthcare Really a System?

The changes rocking the healthcare system are leading towards the development of an organization that will be just that: a system that cares for all people—the sick, the injured, and those seeking to prevent illness or injury—in the most effective way possible. Historically, our healthcare system has not been very systematic in the way it works. It is a fragmented nonsystem, mired in expensive inefficiency and steeped in unnecessarily stressful conditions for patient and worker alike. The creation of the healthcare industry was not based on the ideas of some astute business visionary with a grand plan to delivery optimal healthcare to people. Rather, it emerged over time with its nonsystematized segments and services often in conflict with one another.

By definition, a *system* is a complex but organized whole made up of interrelated and interdependent parts, forming or functioning as a unit. At best, the diverse parts of healthcare, such as inpatient and outpatient care, are certainly interrelated but often not organized. Consider the physician who has cared for a person through years of health and several episodes of illness, and who now requires hospitalization. The system requires that the physician head the team that cares for the hospitalized patient while still managing an office full of patients. This often results in harried visits to the patient early in the morning or late in the evening, while keeping in touch with the hospital staff by phone. In this disorganized and inefficient system, physicians are struggling to maintain the level of competence needed as diagnosis and intervention become increasingly sophisticated and complex. It makes nurse-physician communication difficult at best and leaves vulnerable patients confused.

A new breed of physicians called *hospitalists* are emerging to address this need and challenge the Norman Rockwell image of the "womb-to-tomb" physician who is supposed to function optimally in

> "In a fast-paced, continually shifting environment, resilience to change is the single most important factor that distinguishes those who succeed from those who fail."
>
> —Daryl R. Conner

two places at the same time. As described in a *New York Times* article (March 24, 1998), the hospitalist is an inpatient specialist that takes over for the patient's regular doctor, providing more efficient and continuous care. Because the hospitalist has access to computerized information about the patient's health history, preferences, and advanced directives, the interrelated inpatient and outpatient parts of the health-care system are more seamlessly integrated and the Continuum of Care is maintained more easily.

You may or may not agree with this approach to organize patient care delivery. If this isn't the solution, perhaps others may emerge. The point is that *something* more systematic than what existed before needs to—and will—result from the overhaul of the healthcare industry, and nurses will continue to play an active and vital role. The healthcare system is not just changing, it is being transformed, requiring you to transform as well. Paradigms—the mental maps we use to define, perceive and interpret the world—are shifting, creating new rules to follow, new skills to learn, and new opportunities to seize.

The Riddle of the Lily Pad

When it comes to the workplace, those who say that history is just repeating itself don't have their facts straight. Today we are transforming our relationship to work and to just about everything else as well. While change is not a new experience, the volume, momentum, and complexity of it is different, and it is accelerating faster than ever before. Daryl Conner, author of *Managing at the Speed of Change*, advises his readers to:

> Mark down the date that you read this book. I can say with great confidence that in three years you will look back on this period as "the good old

days" when life was relatively calm. Our world as it is now will look slow and uncomplicated compared to what it is sure to become within the next few years: you have more control and less ambiguity today than you are likely to have for the rest of your life.

To understand the enormity of this and therefore to grasp the impact this kind of change is having on you, Conner asks you to consider the riddle of the lily pad: On day one, a large lake contains only a single, small lily pad. Each day the number of lily pads doubles, until on the 30th day the lake is totally choked with vegetation. On what day is the lake half full?

If you answered day 29, you're right! It takes 29 days for the first half of the lake to fill with lily pads, but only one more day for the lake to become overwhelmed. One moral of the riddle is: Since you can't stop the lily pads (which represent change) from multiplying, you need to expand the lake's capacity (your coping skills) to absorb them.

This is one of the few times in the entire history of the human race in which something so large has happened that it has forever changed all of humankind. Think of the dawning of agriculture, when people were able to conserve their energy by planting crops rather than foraging for food and roaming the land as hunters and gatherers. They used their newfound energy to build cities and governments around the crops, forever changing how life was lived, and heralding a new era for civilization.

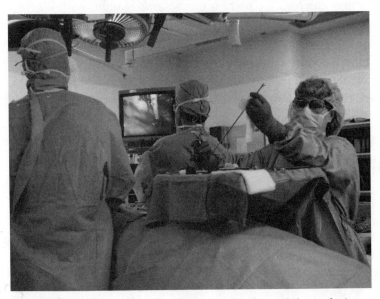

Technological advancements have permanently changed the profession of nursing, requiring nurses to adapt and learn new skills. Keep up with the latest changes, and you will never become obsolete.

Another change, similar in magnitude with today's, was the Industrial Revolution of the late 19th and early 20th centuries, when machinery permitted mass production that resulted in more work opportunities in many different (often skilled) job categories. Unions emerged during this time to protect workers rights. The influence of this era continues to this day.

Today, the emergence of the computer has made data immediately accessible. This increases the capability for instantaneous communication, with the resulting stress of information overload. Those who succeed in this age are the knowledge workers—like nurses, for example—who have access to and know how to use the current and emerging information technologies in their professional and personal lives.

> "Mark down the date that you read this book. I can say with great confidence that in three years you will look back on this period as 'the good old days,' when life was relatively calm. Our world as it is now will look slow and uncomplicated compared to what it is sure to become in the next few years. "You have more control and less ambiguity today than you are likely to have the rest of your life."
> —Daryl Conner, 1992

To use information technologies well means, among other things, to manage the stress inevitably caused as the space and time between knowing something and needing to react to it shortens or disappears. The concept of a margin was developed by Richard Swenson, author of *Margin,* and is described by him as, "The space that once existed in the lives of people who had time to linger over dinner, visit a friend, help the kids with homework, dig in the garden, sleep full nights." The responsibility for managing your margin lies not with the people who affect it from the outside, but rather with you—the person who must live with the margin. Rather than expecting things to slow down or for your employer to provide a more realistic workload, you must create your own margin and develop your own personal strategies for coping.

This issue of margins becomes a rather interesting challenge for the nurse, since it involves the traditional problem of nonassertive submission. This issue has long haunted nurses and turned nursing practice environments into places of passivity where it's difficult to say "no" to unrealistic work assignments and situations. As healthcare restructures its workplace environments, we have an opportunity to transform the behaviors and attitudes that have too long prevented the full use of our voices and contributions.

If you attempt to move into 21st century nursing practice with such antiquated 20th century values as "being all things to all people" and "finishing all your work, perfectly, before you go home," you will find yourself enduring higher levels of self-imposed stress as you are asked to "do more with less," the mandate of some restructuring organizations that cut job positions without necessarily reducing the amount of work. While it is certainly true that the organization has a responsibility to provide reasonable and realistic workloads, it is also true that by agreeing to function in silence while enduring impossible conditions, you are actually perpetuating the dangerous insanity of the situation.

There is a kind of gift inherent in all change: the opportunity to grow, to move beyond previously suffocating restrictions, and—in relation to this example—the ability to say "no," and to establish more reasonable boundaries and limitations. This kind of self-management could also be called self-care, and is a twin partner to clinical nursing skills. Self-care is also one of the legs of the three-legged stool representing a balanced nursing practice. It is key to your personal and professional well-being, and as an antidote to burnout, it should not be underestimated or ignored.

Chapter 3

The Nurse Pioneer

Frontier: 1—The outer edges of a settled territory. 2—A territory in which pursuits, activities, and interests are confined. 3—A geographical region between two countries. 4—A domain, a province.

> "Life is either a daring adventure or nothing."
> —Helen Keller

It is clear that the Healthcare Revolution presents challenges to patients, nurses, and all healthcare workers as they find themselves exploring territories where systems are unfamiliar, policies are destablizing, and roles and relationships are reforming. For patients, this new frontier means getting used to a new cast of characters who act as gatekeepers to restrict and regulate their use of healthcare services in newly emerged territories along the Continuum of Care. These territories include transitional hospitals, subacute centers or, even more often, the home. As nurses, we find ourselves in pioneering roles as we enter new work scenarios along the outer edges of healthcare's frontier while exploring the outer edges of our own comfort zones, as well.

Comparing the definition of a frontier with some typical experiences resulting from the Healthcare Revolution sheds some light on what is unfolding.

A Frontier Is a Domain, a Province

In this new frontier, nurse pioneers are discovering ways to enlarge the domains and provinces of nursing practice beyond previously limiting frameworks and into such expanded "territories" as nurse practitioner, nurse case manager, and nurse informatics specialist.

A Frontier Is a Geographical Region Between Two Countries

The geographical region between the two "countries" of acute care and postacute care has become a country now known as the Continuum of Care, with such emerging territories as transitional hospitals, subacute centers, and psychiatric home care.

A Frontier Describes the Outer Edges of a Settled Territory

This could describe nurses in the new Informatics territories, or the newly expanded territories of the nurse manager and nurse executive who are leading the reengineering efforts of many healthcare organizations, or the nurse who provides consulting services to these organizations, perhaps regarding work redesign. Consider, as well, the new territories of nurse entrepreneurs who establish clinics run by nurses, or those who open home care agencies.

A Frontier Has Unfamiliar Geography with Indistinct Boundaries, Requiring Maps for Ease of Travel

New career and workplace maps are needed by all nurses, novice and expert alike, as we move around healthcare's restructured territories. In addition, the indistinct boundaries between nurse practitioners and physicians who are both primary care providers present a challenge not unlike what the pioneers of the Old West faced in trying to preserve what they had while forging into new lands. Nurse practitioners must work to maintain the distinction between the disciplines of nursing and medicine, preserving their separate missions (of caring and curing, respectively) while at the same time developing "maps" to decrease role confusion for the healthcare community. In this way they can fulfill what Linda Peavy, in a book called *Frontier Women*, describes as the challenge of women pioneers, namely to "hold on to the roots of their past, yet adapt to the changes and challenges of the present and the future."

Just as pioneers in the west helped to chart new territory, nurse pioneers of today have the opportunity to participate in creating a freer, more democratic nursing workplace. However, in this quest for a more equitable balance of power; we must try not to repeat a great failure of our pioneer ancestors; namely, their inability to exist side by side with those who were in the territory first, the Native Americans. Finding ways to overcome differences through interdependence and collaboration should be a goal for everyone in healthcare's new territories.

The Nurse Pioneer

> **Pioneer:** 1—An explorer, an investigator, a prospector. 2—One who originates or helps open a new line of activity, an early settler.

Just like our pioneer ancestors, you too have the opportunity to explore, investigate, prospect, and settle new territories in today's healthcare environment while learning to think and act differently within them. As a nurse pioneer, you can develop characteristics like our ancestors, including the ability to:

- Live along the outer edges of your comfort zone, where physical and emotional tension are the companions of growth and forward progress.
- Bounce back from the unexpected, often discovering that the unexpected creates interesting, if unplanned adventures.
- Adapt with flexibility to unforeseen circumstances, shifting your goals, priorities, and activities as necessary.
- Travel lightly, leaving behind excess baggage (often in the form of outdated values and limiting beliefs) so that there is enough room for what's new and what's next.

- Persist tenaciously in the pursuit of your professional and personal goals, refusing to give up easily.
- Know how to "think outside of a box," meaning to find or invent new and creative solutions to old problems, on your own as well as collaboratively. This often involves forging new relationships, creating new pathways of possibilities, and freeing yourself of attitudes and behaviors that have the potential to constrain or dull your sense of adventure.

A good book that illustrates this last characteristic is Frank A. Prince's *C and the Box: A Paradigm Parable.* In this little volume, Prince conveys the value of leaving your comfortable "box" of familiar habits through a series of cartoons showing C—a letter of the alphabet given life as a character in a story—finding a way to overcome professional malaise through creativity and invention. C eventually learns to enjoy this newfound discovery and goes on to show other characters how to benefit from it. You can, too.

To continue the pioneer metaphor, nurses rely on each other for support and information, and like their pioneer ancestors they:

Considering yourself a nurse pioneer on a new frontier of healthcare is one way to thrive in restructured workplaces.

- Send out scouts to determine the trends and predictions that will influence the healthcare workplace
- Circle their wagons to unite against professional threats to their well-being
- Hold "pow-wows" to coach and mentor one another
- Tell stories around the campfire to inspire and reinforce the pioneer spirit

Of course, whether you consider yourself a nurse pioneer or a nurse in the "time of the parentheses" may matter less than knowing that the change you are witnessing and experiencing is not only irrevocable, but will continue and even increase in its depth, duration, and intensity. There are many metaphors to describe what is changing in healthcare and the effects those changes will have on your life as a nurse. These will surely be the worst of times for those unable to embrace the changes ahead. Likewise, you can transform them into the best of times if you are willing to seize the opportunities within it. President Bill Clinton's words are helpful here: "The important question of our time is whether we can make change our friend, not our enemy."

Chapter 4

Maintaining Balance and Strength During Times of Change

To secure a place for yourself in 21st century healthcare, you need to focus on three components of your worklife: Your clinical and professional competencies, your career development skills, and your stress management strategies.

> "The first chore in managing change is the toughest: self-management. Handle that right and you're halfway home."
>
> —Price Pritchett

Clinical and professional competencies include your educational credentials, work experience, cross-trained skills, and professional certification. Career development skills include knowing how to market yourself effectively; for example, using your résumé to advertise and highlight your nursing expertise, successfully selling yourself to a potential employer in an interview, and networking for information and support. Stress management skills are required to cope with the constant change and permanent transition typical today.

Remember the three-legged stool from chapter 1? Think of these three components as comprising one of each of the legs on your three-legged stool. While the focus of this book is mostly on the career strategy leg of your worklife, information is presented about how the changes in healthcare will affect the professional/clinical leg. In addition, integrated throughout the book are tips and guidelines about how to strengthen the stress management leg, with additional resources provided in this book's appendix.

Self Care: Stress Management You Can Count On

When situations change, an area of focus that is often neglected is *you* and what you need to do to strengthen your ability to manage the stress that naturally accompanies change. By strengthening this ability, you can sustain yourself through the transition to what will be next. This is especially important if the change is unwelcome, unexpected, or is something which you may not be in agreement with. You may have a limited influence on what will happen around you, but you always have a degree of control over yourself and your responses to it. Through self-management you can reassess your needs, set new goals, sustain your well-being, and inhibit feeling victimized or powerless. Ongoing self-management in the face of constant change can become a source of personal fuel to propel you towards what is best for you while taking full advantage of the opportunities change brings.

This kind of self-focus may be new to you if you've been traditionally educated and socialized to be other-focused. That can make it hard for you to adjust. As good as many nurses are in meeting the physical, emotional, mental, and spiritual needs of others, when it comes to applying this knowledge to themselves, they are sometimes rather ineffective. This shows up in different ways for different nurses. For example, if you work for 8, 10, or 12 hours without a meal break, you are not meeting your physical needs for nutrition, hydration, and rest. Another example is when you are unable to say no to the requests of others, even if it entails unreasonable work assignments. Leaving this kind of self-focus out of the self-other equation is not good nursing practice. It is certainly not good for you, and while your intentions may be good, it doesn't benefit the patient either. If you are out of touch with your basic needs, you make a poor role model and you put your patients at risk. This kind of behavior is also a perfect setup for feeling victimized and for perpetual stress and eventual burnout.

To determine the degree of difficulty you may have in the ability to focus on your needs while tending to the needs of others, consider the following situation. Imagine you are traveling on an airplane with a three-year-old child who is totally dependent on you for his safety and well-being. Now imagine that, after enjoying a meal, you and this child have drifted off to sleep only to be awakened by the lights flashing on and off in the cabin, the plane rocking back and forth, and unusual sounds coming from somewhere under the floor of the plane. As you try to figure out what is happening, the oxygen masks drop from the overhead compartments and the captain is now announcing you must put them on. Whose mask do you put on first, yours or the child's?

If you answered yours, you are right. No matter what is happening—no matter how frightened, needy, and demanding the child may be—it is quite likely that you will both become unconscious quickly if you tend to the needs of the child first. True, he will not know how to put the mask on without your help . . . but if the child struggles because he is panicking or because he doesn't understand what is happening, precious time will be lost. While your instincts may tell you to see to your needs last, those instincts must be inhibited to insures the child's safety as well as your own.

In the same way, by attempting to work without "oxygen"—rest breaks, assertive communication, and appropriate boundaries—you are potentially impairing your own well-being as well as those you care for and work with. This kind of stress management could also be called self care and has three major components: self-awareness, self-management, and self-renewal. Self-awareness refers to the capacity you have to look inward for understanding and clarification, to learn from experience, to understand the meaning an experience is having for you and also to understand how you may be influencing others. Self-management involves the strategies and skills you develop to respond to life situations in ways that achieve your personal and interpersonal goals and sustain your well-being. Time management, conflict resolution, assertive communication are examples of self-management strategies. Self-renewal refers to ways in which you preserve, enhance, and restore the energy required for your personal and professional life through the use of regular routines that reduce or neutralize the effects of stress. Self-renewal strategies include eating for high energy, maintaining physical fitness, and meditation.

By practicing these three components of self care diligently as you develop your professional and clinical skills and career strategies, you will guide yourself through the ongoing changes in healthcare and will have stress management strategies that you can count on. The quiz on the following page is reprinted by permission of *Nursing Spectrum*. Use it to determine your ability to use some selected self care strategies that are essential to letting the future in.

Let the Future In

Check the boxes of the statements that apply to you, add up your points, and see how you rate according to the key at the bottom.

❏ I work along the outer edges of my comfort zone. I seek out new experiences even if or especially because they make me edgy. My life has informed risks and challenges built into it. (5 points)

❏ I practice proactivity rather than reactivity. I build and match my transferable skills to marketplace needs. I change before I have to. (4 points)

❏ I manage my margin (the space between my limit and my overload). I use the word *no* in measured doses and assertive ways. I maintain flexibly firm interpersonal boundaries. (4 points)

❏ I am online. I am growing comfortable with computers and the use of the Internet for electronic networking, support, and information. (3 points)

❏ I deflect doom and gloom. I surround myself with people who are hopeful and optimistic. I know how to immunize myself against the contagion of pessimists and nay-sayers. (4 points)

If you scored 16 to 20: Congratulations! You get the message, but don't be lulled into complacency.

If you scored 11 to 15: Good work! However, you can reach still higher.

If you scored 6 to 10: Take care! You may be hoping to recreate the past rather than allow the future in.

If you scored 0 to 5: Watch out! You are in danger of being blown away by the winds of change.

Living and Working Along the Outer Edges of Your Comfort Zone

Hanging on to familiar routines, skills and relationships in an effort to protect yourself from the discomfort that naturally accompanies a new experience is one of the most self-defeating things you could do during these fluid times of change. By resisting change this way, you will paradoxically create the very experience you are trying to prevent, and wind up with even less control and more stress. Here's an equation to remember: change equals stress. And a degree of stress is required for motivation, momentum, and even the ability to support your body while you stand.

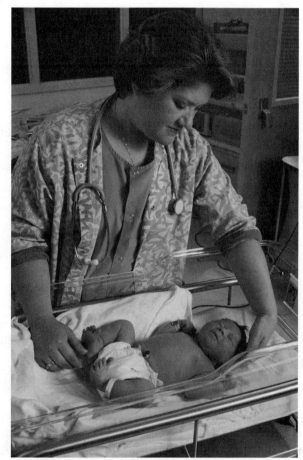

Nurses in all clinical areas (not just pediatrics) need to decide what constitutes a worthwhile challenge.

You have two choices here. You can either put your head in the sand, hoping the predictions of ever-accelerating change are wrong, or you can strengthen yourself for the inevitable by learning how to move in and out of your comfort zone.

For example, Doris knew that moving from the pediatric ICU to the neonatal ICU scared her, and for that very reason, she knew she had to do it. She recognized that her comfort where she was could lull her into a dangerous complacency. She saw the potential discomfort of the transfer as a challenge, and was also wise enough to know how the experience would increase her present and future employability.

This same nurse could contemplate leaving her comfort zone again when the neonatal ICU eventually becomes familiar and comfortable. She is exercising her change management muscles by developing more resilience and flexibility. In what ways can you challenge yourself? Take on more risk?

Practice Proactivity

Proactive nurses are those who watch marketplace trends and work toward developing the transferable skills required. They are self-starters who take their responsibility for self management seriously. They know that this is the path to 21st century career security and the replacement for 20th century job security.

An example is the nurse who volunteers to be part of a work redesign committee in a restructuring organization. Not only will she obtain direct information, bypassing the stress of relying on rumor-mill distortions for information, but she can reap the added benefit of helping to shape her future work responsibilities. Where can proactivity enhance your life? In what ways can you practice it?

Manage Your Margin

As discussed before, your margin is the space between you and a situation or a person that has the potential to stretch you beyond your limits. It's a gap. It is your reserve. It's the difference between your limit and your load, and is the opposite of overload. The Age of Information is creating smaller and smaller margins between what you need done and your ability to do it. Many of us do more than one thing so routinely that it seems almost boring to do only one thing at a time.

A few tips for managing your margins are:

- Learn to say no. This takes careful consideration and often a reappraisal of values in current workplaces, where many nurses are being asked to do more with less. Separating assertive communication from resistance to change is essential here.

- Sustain your physical well-being. Differentiate between eating for energy and eating for pleasure; make sure you exercise enough and don't think of sleep as a disposable commodity.
- Take time management seriously. Instead of only prioritizing your schedule, commit yourself to scheduling your priorities, professional *and* personal. If workouts are actually written into your daily agenda book, you'll be much more like to do it.
- Push back the technological invasions into your life. Control when and if you want others to have immediate and instant access to you through fax machines, beepers, and cell phones.

Get Online

As a 21st century nurse, you know that being online means using the Internet for personal and professional networking, support, and information. You may not be a computer maven, but you can integrate computers into your life in a variety of ways.

Employers are becoming less and less interested in nurses who refuse to enter the electronic age and who might be even more foolish by joking about how computer-illiterate they are.

Ways of using the Internet include exploring employment and job opportunity sites, researching clinical information, and networking with colleagues through e-mail and chat rooms.

Oprah Winfrey wrote a weight-loss book entitled *Make the Connection*. What needs to happen for you to make the connection and enter this exciting electronic experience essential to your 21st century nursing career? What small step can you take?

Deflect Doom and Gloom

Fear of change, inaccurate information, and unresolved emotional difficulties are the basis for the doom and gloom some nurses seem to perpetuate. Separate yourself from and immunize your self against those nurses who have an endless need to whine, complain, and act like victims by:

- Getting information from reliable sources rather than the rumor mill. Ask questions, read, attend seminars.
- Surrounding yourself with people who are optimistic as well as realistic and hopeful about life in general and about the healthcare workplace specifically.
- Refusing to engage in doom and gloom conversations. Set limits. Leave the room if necessary.
- Considering new relationships if all else fails. Some people need more help to change than you may be able to provide.

Self-care strategies are woven and embedded throughout this book. Seek them out and use them.

Chapter 5

For the Newly Graduated Nurse

Welcome to nursing! You are embarking on a career whose challenge and diversity will provide you with some of the finest opportunities for professional achievement and personal growth to be found anywhere. You are also entering the healthcare industry at a time of unprecedented upheaval as well as expanded opportunity. While this is certainly a confusing time, it is also an exciting time . . . a time when some of the old ways restricting and inhibiting the value of nursing in the eyes of many (sometimes even the nurse) are beginning to fade away and to be replaced with an ever growing recognition of our worth and our contribution to the health and well-being of those we care for. It is this positive perception of the changes in healthcare that can shape your purpose in nursing, sustain you through the challenges inherent in it, and provide you with the professional satisfaction you are seeking.

In many ways, the kind of experience you will have as a nurse will be up to you. In nursing, as in life, attitude is everything. So much of life, including your life as a nurse, is about attitude—what you think about what you see and how to purposefully shape it into something meaningful to you. Some tips that will assist you in shaping your experience follow. Use these tips along with the information in this book to launch yourself into nursing practice and keep yourself on track.

Deflect Doom and Gloom Thinking and Ignore Pessimistic Thinkers.

Infuse yourself with the energy of those who believe in the possible. Separate from those who seem habituated to the impossible.

Find a Mentor or Coach.

Nursing practice can be as complicated as it is rewarding. Mentors and coaches can be stabilizing forces of encouraging direction.

Establish a Peer Support Group.

Select people who are willing to speak to your strengths, support your growth, and search for solutions. Take care to prevent this useful strategy from disintegrating into nonproductive, contagious, and energy-depleting gripe sessions. Find a facilitator, if necessary, or rotate this function among the participants.

Prepare for Reality Shock.

All new graduates in all industries, especially professionals, need to allow time to merge school values with work realities. Being prepared for this necessary stage of professional development will ease the difficulty of this transition.

Resist Being "Eaten" by Your "Elders."

There is a terrible saying in nursing: "Nurses eat their young." You may have even experienced a little of this as a student, when some nurses might have been less receptive or helpful to you than they should have been. Prepare yourself for this potential by developing assertive communication, seeking out mentors and peer support, and trusting in yourself.

Clarify Your Values.

Resist internalizing an implicit set of impossible-to-meet values that are never spoken aloud or taught but which you might find yourself mindlessly enacting. This value, enforced by peer pressure, infers that nurses are "all things to all people, and need to finish all their work, on time, perfectly before they go home." Think about it: All things? All people? All their work? Perfectly? Refute it! Resist it! Clarify and operate by a more realistic set of standards that recognizes the 24-hour nature of a team-based model of practice. Once again, seek out supportive mentors, coaches, and peers.

Be Patient with Yourself, Even if Others Are Not.

It will take time for you to move from a novice nurse to a proficient one. Your education gives you the basic foundation and sketches an outline upon which you will build from the time you graduate, throughout your entire career.

Believe in Yourself and What You Have to Offer.

New graduates, especially those with a B.S.N., have a competitive edge and should use it. Market yourself effectively. Your eagerness, fresh idealism, and willingness to learn is a very attractive commodity to organizations often mired in resistance to change.

Define your nursing mission/purpose and develop a vision of your work as a nurse. Chapter 7, "Product Development," will help you explore why and how you need to do this. Your mission and vision will contribute to your inner and career stability as you move between workplaces more often than generations of nurses that preceded you. It will ensure that you have satisfying work that has a potential to fulfill you rather than burn you out.

Find Your Niche.

There are many ways to be a nurse and something for everyone in nursing. See chapter 8, "Marketplace Research," to explore the many roles and venues in nursing along healthcare's expanding Continuum of Care.

Take your responsibility for self care seriously. Care for yourself as well as you are learning to care for others. Follow the advice of Gloria Steinem who said to read the Golden Rule in both directions: Do unto others as you would have them do unto you (this is the part with which we are familiar). And, remember to do unto yourself as well as you do unto others.

PART TWO

The Business of You, Inc.

Chapter 6

Your Career Is a Business

William Bridges, author of a book entitled *Job Shift: How to Prosper in a Workplace Without Jobs*, advises workers everywhere to convert themselves into a business by "seeing yourself as a self-contained economic entity, not as a component part looking for a whole within which you can (hopefully) function."

> "I have failed many times."
> —Henry Ford, in response to the question, "To what do you attribute your success?"

The following list of points expands on his advice to develop a self-employed attitude in a transformed job market, whether you are an employee, a consultant, a supplier, or an entrepreneur. You can do wonders towards changing your career by:

- Being "vendor-minded" (in the case of nursing, this would translate into being "consumer-oriented")
- Seeing yourself surrounded by a market, whether or not you are on the payroll of an organization
- Joining—not blindly working for—your organization and customers (patients)
- Thinking like an entrepreneur, or in the case of the employed nurse, an *intrapreneur*, by identifying or creating work opportunities
- Integrating independence with interdependence: relying on yourself and collaborating with others
- Finding new and creative ways to contribute your competencies in new marketplaces, including the ones that exist within your present place of employment.

- Committing to continuous learning.
- Replacing your fears about work with creating meaningful work, believing you have a contribution to make.
- Beginning the process of change with yourself, your own personal growth.

Bridges advocates a whole new way of looking at work and at employment, even if you don't change the location of your workplace. He is describing a real paradigm shift, a way to reframe, to think differently about something you may have always done and many of you will continue doing, namely your work.

Bridges is not a lone voice in a seemingly unconventional world of workplace reframing. *U.S. News and World Report,* a very conventional, Main Street USA publication, devoted 32 pages in 1996 to an article entitled, "You, Inc." The article describes how all United States industries, including healthcare, "have leapt headlong into the information age, and how careers will never be the same. . . . At no time in modern history have so many workers been so totally reliant on their own wits and resources to thrive. . . . The upshot: You, Inc. may be the fastest growing employment segment in the economy, as people learn to invest in themselves as if they *were* a corporation."

A primary mission of You, Inc. is to continuously explore the answer to the following question: How is your service—what you have to offer—at least as good or perhaps even better than the same or similar nursing "businesses" of others? If you, along with 50 other nurses, apply for the job of medical-surgical staff nurse, for example, what makes you at least as qualified, or even more qualified?

Another variation of the question above is: What value would you add to the mission of the organization where you are seeking employment (or where you are currently working) as compared to the others also seeking it or working within it? In what ways do you or have you improved the quality of service that the organization provides, over and above the minimum requirement of showing up for work and performing the tasks required in the job description? If a particular activity (a nursing job function or role, for example) is not adding value, if it cannot somehow be translated into direct or indirect profit, it cannot continue unchanged if the organization is to survive. Harsh as this may sound, this kind of thinking does not have to be mutually exclusive from caring for and about patients, or those who take care of them. More and more, it is seen as the *way* to care, as long as it is tempered with sound ethical and moral stan-

THE NURSE WHO CAN COMPETE MOST EFFECTIVELY

Professional Experience

- Possesses targeted, progressive, cumulative work experience as a generalist and a specialist
- Can articulate examples of "value-added" work experiences
- Is aware of, able to support, and can contribute to patient-focused care in a consumer-oriented business environment
- Has transferable skills
- Is cross-trained
- Seeks continuing education
- Becomes computer literate and Internet savvy
- Earns the Bachelor of Science in Nursing
- Pursues advanced educational preparation commensurate with career goals
- Receives ANCC board-certification as a generalist, specialist, or other professional certification)
- Seeks professional membership

Personal Characteristics

- Is flexible, adaptive, assertive, confident, empowered
- Is self-directed and team-oriented
- Strives to be an innovative problem solver
- Does not accept status quo
- Is willing to take risks
- Learns from mistakes
- Resolves conflicts
- Thinks critically
- Is a master networker

Note: This is not a complete list, but rather some examples that contribute to effective professional practice and employment in a competitive healthcare marketplace. Feel free to add to the list, personalizing it to your situation.

dards applied to patient care as well as employment practices. Since this is a reality in the healthcare marketplace, it needs to be a reality for You, Inc. as well.

To compete most effectively, you should know the ways in which your product is different from others', have examples of those differences in your professional portfolio, and be assertive enough to state them. You should get as close as you can to having the professional experiences and personal characteristics listed below. You should have a plan for those that you don't have yet, knowing that you are a work in progress in need of the same kind of continuous quality improvement as the healthcare organizations you may work for. To get what you want, you must know how to stand out so you don't fade out.

The healthcare workplace has new rules of engagement, so to speak, for all of its customers, patients and nurses alike. As the rules of the game have changed, so should you. Becoming the chief executive officer of You, Inc. allows you to play the game by these new rules and also create some of your own. If you think this is a far-fetched idea, an interesting philosophy without practicality, compare the business functions of You, Inc. with the more conventional organizations with which you are familiar:

Organizations and Corporations	**You, Inc.**
Have a mission statement, a clearly stated purpose	Has a mission statement aligned with values and a mission
Have an operating license	Has an RN license, and perhaps others
Are insured against malpractice and accidental injury claims	Carries malpractice insurance and other insurance as indicated
Operate based on written standards of practice	Utilizes ANA Standards in the practice of nursing
Abide by ethical standards	Abides by the ANA Code of Ethics
Utilize policies and procedures for the delivery of its services and the fulfillment of its mission	Utilizes policies and procedures that determine where, when, and for how long You, Inc. will provide its services in a particular segment of the healthcare marketplace

Engage in continuous quality improvement programs	Engages in continuous training and education to improve the quality and marketability of skills and services
Seek and apply for recognition by associations and accrediting agencies for outstanding achievement and excellence in service, such as Magnet Hospital Status awarded by ANCC	Seeks out recognition for professional achievement through ANCC board certification, or through other professional associations
Builds alliances, coalitions, networks, and partnerships with other organizations	Considers itself a partner to healthcare organizations. The organization has patients that need healthcare services. You, Inc. provides those services and builds professional and personal networks.
Competes effectively with other organizations that provide the same service by means of effective marketing and public relations strategies	Utilizes business strategies to compete effectively, including product development, marketplace research, advertising (résumé), sales (interviewing), networking, and the development of a marketing plan.

As you compare the two lists, you may recognize that most of the expectations and functions described for You, Inc. aren't too different from what is expected of nurses who want career excellence, except perhaps for the last item about utilizing business strategies to compete effectively. And that's where You, Inc. comes in; this is its founding purpose. The chapters that follow will help you explore some of the You, Inc. business skills needed to be a nurse pioneer in the emerging territories of the new healthcare marketplace. Imagine yourself as the chief executive officer and chief operating officer of You, Inc., situated in some centralized place, your own "nursing office," if you will, perhaps a headquarters of operation in your home. From this place you can plan, implement, and track the activities of You Inc. as well as oversee and coordinate the following You, Inc. "departments":

You, Inc. Department	Department Responsibilities and Functions
Product Development	In charge of developing and articulating who you are and what you have to offer, including your mission statement, values and needs, vision, and preferred nursing roles and competencies
Marketplace Research	Conducts ongoing research and makes recommendations about where along the Continuum of Care what you have to offer is most needed
Advertising	Creates and revises your résumé and maintains your professional portfolio
Sales	Develops and hones techniques for interviewing and selling your nursing skills and competencies
Networking	Creates and maintains professional and personal alliances and relationships
Marketing Plan	Performs ongoing assessments of needs and develops strategic career plans with defined goals, stated tasks, and specific timelines

Debbie, a single parent of a two-year-old daughter, demonstrates some of how You, Inc. can work. She is a fee-for-service (per diem) home-care nurse who works for several home-care agencies simultaneously. She pays for her own and her daughter's health and disability insurance and has recently established a private retirement fund managed by a financial advisor at her local bank.

She is an ANCC-certified, medical-surgical nurse practicing at the generalist level and will soon complete an adult nurse practitioner program paid for by scholarships, savings targeted for starting school, and one low-interest loan. The work she does at the home-care agencies is aligned with one of her most cherished values, independence, and supports her mission of tending to the physical and emotional health of geriatric patients. Her long-term vision is to create more in-home mental health services, especially for the isolated home-bound patient that makes up the majority of her practice and for which very little mobile support is available.

Debbie arranges her work schedule and maintains an adequate income so that it best supports her school goals and parenting responsibilities by reducing the number of hours she is available to the agencies when school is in session, and increasing them during semester breaks. She is careful about the kind of assignments she accepts when she is in school, choosing lighter assignments such as home health aide supervisions which require less of a long-term commitment than carrying her own caseload of patients. Debbie self-manages the components of work life traditionally managed by employers, including health and disability insurance, retirement savings, tuition reimbursement, time scheduling, and patient assignments. She carries her own malpractice insurance. She misses the natural relationship-building that goes on in workplaces where people are in the same building all day, but substitutes school-based involvement when classes are in session and tries to attend professional meetings during semester breaks.

Debbie relishes the freedom that accompanies this style of working, and she asks her more risk-averse peers to consider the alternative: The "safety" of traditional employment in exchange for less control over professional direction, and not being able to create the kind of work schedule that allows her to enjoy school and spend time with her daughter.

Empowerment

In some ways, there are really *two* revolutions going on in healthcare: One is about the structure of the industry itself, and the other is about the shift in the thinking and behavior of the people in it. Nurses, like employees everywhere, are beginning to recognize the value of freeing themselves from the mindset of a limiting employee mentality and adopting a more liberated self-employed attitude. Whether those with this self-employed attitude continue working for others or choose to work for themselves matters less than their change of consciousness about the work they do. The most important part of the self-employed attitude is the recognition of who "owns" the work being done.

The contract between employer and employee that originated in the Industrial Revolution is no longer valid: It now contributes to potentially dysfunctional employment relationships and the mistaken belief that job security is guaranteed in return for loyalty to the organization. In its place has risen a mutual interdependence in which both the employer and the employee maintain a relationship with each other for as long as the relationship is financially profitable and professionally useful. This new psychological employment contract has important implications for nursing career paths, and has been well-described by David Noer, author of *Healing the Wounds*, as follows:

Old Employment Contract

- Tenure and long-term relationships
- Linear promotion as reward for performance, within fixed job descriptions
- Lifetime employment through loyalty to the organization, which provides long-term career paths and discourages external hiring

This approach resulted in a workforce that was older, nondiverse, plateaued, demotivated, codependent, and mediocre.

New Employment Contract

- Employment is situational with flexible, portable benefit plans
- Blurred distinction between full-time, part-time, and temporary employees
- Reward for performance is tenure-free acknowledgement of contribution achieved through self-directed work teams and nonhierarchical performance systems
- Employees are more autonomous and not "taken care of" long term
- Loyalty means responsibility and good work within nontraditional career paths

This approach can result in a workforce that is flexible, motivated, task invested, empowered, and responsible. While not all organizations have fully embraced the new structure described here, they are moving in that direction, and therefore so should the nurse.

The Empowerment Continuum

To be empowered is to act on your own behalf. To stay loyal to yourself, our needs, values, mission and vision while committing yourself to the goals of the organization for the time you are there. See the chart on the next page:

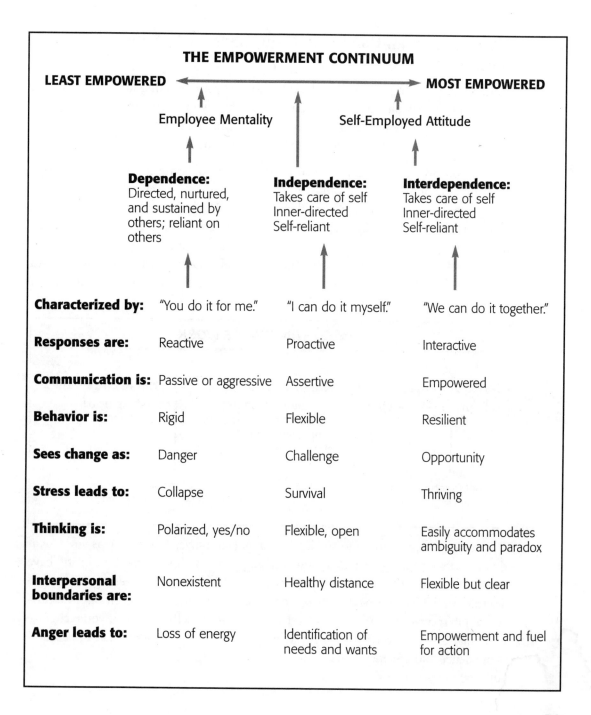

THE EMPOWERMENT CONTINUUM

LEAST EMPOWERED ⟵————————————⟶ MOST EMPOWERED

Employee Mentality   Self-Employed Attitude

Dependence: Directed, nurtured, and sustained by others; reliant on others

Independence: Takes care of self Inner-directed Self-reliant

Interdependence: Takes care of self Inner-directed Self-reliant

Characterized by:	"You do it for me."	"I can do it myself."	"We can do it together."
Responses are:	Reactive	Proactive	Interactive
Communication is:	Passive or aggressive	Assertive	Empowered
Behavior is:	Rigid	Flexible	Resilient
Sees change as:	Danger	Challenge	Opportunity
Stress leads to:	Collapse	Survival	Thriving
Thinking is:	Polarized, yes/no	Flexible, open	Easily accommodates ambiguity and paradox
Interpersonal boundaries are:	Nonexistent	Healthy distance	Flexible but clear
Anger leads to:	Loss of energy	Identification of needs and wants	Empowerment and fuel for action

Shifting from an Employee Mentality to a Self-Employed Attitude

To develop a self-employed attitude, two shifts in your thinking are necessary. The first is a reconceptualization of the manner in which you work and where it falls on The Continuum of Work, and the second is a rethinking of who owns the *work* you do (as opposed to the *job* you have); to whom does your work belong?

Think about work as existing on a continuum, with full-time employment, perhaps for a lifetime, on one end, and full-time self-employment on the extreme other end. Both of these ways of working have always existed. Either you work for someone else or you work for yourself. Someplace in the middle is shorter-term, project-based work, perhaps with multiple and/or simultaneous employers. This model will be more prevalent as we move forward. The more comfortable you are moving back and forth along this continuum, the more secure and interesting your career will be.

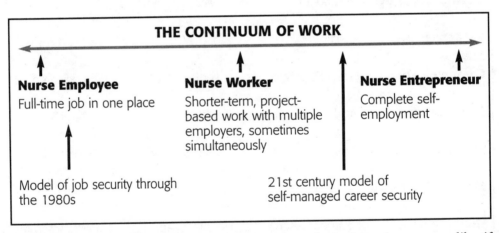

Of course, you can choose to work for only one employer for as long as you like, if that is mutually advantageous to both you and your employer. But you can still have a self-employed attitude because your skills, abilities, and talents belong to you and are transferable to your next work option. There's a difference between career security and job security, and there is a wonderful freedom in self-reliance. If you recognize that what exists between you and your employer is interdependence, as opposed to dependence and codependence, your career is already well on its way to becoming your own personal business.

Chapter 7

Product Development

Specifying and Strengthening Who You Are and What You Have to Offer

> "The first thing you have to do before you find the treasure is to find the map."
> —Barbara Sher

There are two components of product development, each deserving your attention and needing to carry equal weight. The first component is about your pro-
fessional nursing life, and the second is the personal side of your life which, while it should be separate, still greatly influences and is influenced by your professional life. Your wholeness and integrity during these times of constant change and permanent transition rely heavily on your ability to nurture, strengthen, and develop both aspects of your identity, professional and personal. These two aspects are inextricably woven together despite any attempt to separate them, whether on your part or by some other circumstance, such as workplace traditions and values. The workplace axiom of "leave your problems at home" speaks to the necessary but only temporary separation of the professional and the personal aspects of your life. It's a way to triage experiences in order to allow for effective focus, such as, "Right now, I'm taking care of this patient. Later, I'll decide what to do about my financial problems." At some point, both require equal attention.

Another reason why both the professional and personal areas of your life require a measured equality of attention is the relevance this experience has to the nurse-patient relationship, the most sacred and revered component of nursing practice. Clearly, the uniqueness, strength, and expression of your personal self-influences the quality and effectiveness of this important relationship, which is not only responsible for facilitating healing in the patient, but also contributes to your professional satisfaction and growth.

A focus on personal development is also essential for you to establish, strengthen, and communicate your limits and boundaries, the margins between what you can and cannot do safely and ethically in the "do more with less" environments typical of healthcare today.

Attention to the personal side of product development will also result in the emergence of the work behaviors that employers want in the new workplace of healthcare, namely, flexibility, assertiveness, empowerment, independent and collaborative behaviors, and risk taking.

All experts who speak about the changing world of work and what it takes to be in it, point repeatedly to the need for a self-focus. Cliff Hakim, author of *We Are All Self-Employed*, says to "begin the process of change with yourself." In 1996, *U.S. News and World Report* advised readers to "invest in yourself, in your own personal growth, as if you were a corporation."

The theme of taking responsibility for your personal growth and its influence on your professional life is woven throughout this book, implicitly and explicitly. These twin partners of your nursing practice, the professional and the personal, are two sides of the same coin: One represents the care of others, the other represents the care of the self. Despite the obvious necessity for this dual focus, self-care for the nurse is not as dominant an issue in nursing education or in nursing practice as it needs to be. While the reasons for this are numerous (see the appendix for excellent discussions and further information), these times of liberating change provide not only the opportunity but the necessity to focus on the personal side of the coin, and shatter the oppressive notion that self-care skills should not receive the equal and formal attention that professional and clinical skills have long received.

In this product development section, you will have an opportunity to explore selected components relevant to your professional as well as your personal development.

Consider this information a modest overview of a much more vast terrain. Allow it to point you in the direction of a deeper exploration.

Self-Awareness During Times Of Permanent Transition

Permanent transition, the need to continuously adapt to something new during times of constant change, is a fact of life at the dawn of this new century. Recognizing this will prevent you from losing your competitive edge as the health-care marketplace continues to shift. You can expect a marketplace shift significant enough to dramatically alter your professional or personal life to occur about every six months. To adjust, you will need to determine, by means of a self-initiated, biannual review, whether what you have to offer in the form of your "product"(your professional and clinical skills) is still in alignment with your current job responsibilities, and with your life in general.

Confronted with this scenario, you have two options. The first is to take your product to an employment situation where it is needed more. The second is to realign your product with your current employment situation as it changes. One way to discover the best option for you is to continually observe how your abilities relate to your current or potential employer's.

What cannot be emphasized enough is that your review needs to be *self-initiated*, and that it should occur at least *biannually,* or more aptly, be *ongoing.* Drop the ball here and you may have a prescription for greater career distress than necessary. Stay alert for signals in your place of employment that indicate a need to activate a career move, whether within your current workplace or elsewhere. While the hiring of outside reengineering consultants is the most obvious indicator, other signs to watch for include the following list adapted from *Texas Nursing 1995* and *The Oregon Nurse, 1995:*

- Changes in patient census with a trend that indicate lower numbers as compared to previous years and to industry standards
- Changes in staffing patterns leading to staff shortages, including hiring freezes, the elimination of positions following staff resignation, delays in filling vacancies, increased use of agency personnel, frequent floating of staff between units, increases in part time positions with a corresponding decrease in full-

time positions, and an increased trend toward early retirement and buyouts for senior staff

- Changes in the readiness and availability of supplies and services of outside vendors
- Increased use of outside consultants for training, especially cross-training
- Any trend towards changing the nursing skill mix to a lower percentage of RN's and a higher percentage of ancillary staff such as the cross training of RN staff to other nursing specialties and to non-nursing clinical tasks, the cross-training of professional and ancillary staff to cover other hospital departments, and an increasing trend of using ancillary staff to perform tasks previously done exclusively by RNs
- Consolidation of management services and reduction of overall management layers
- Elimination of preferential staffing and scheduling systems, i.e., the 12-hour/ 3-day per week work schedule preferred by many nurses is replaced by the traditional eight hour/five day per week schedule
- Reduced hours of operation for ancillary and support departments such as pharmacy with a corresponding shift of responsibility to the nursing units
- Decreases in the overall benefits packages

A lot of what you need to know about finding career satisfaction and moving around effectively in today's job market is contained in the answers to following questions:

- Who are you?
- What do you have to offer?
- Who needs it?

In this chapter, will explore the answers to the first two questions. The third question will be explored in chapter 8, "Marketplace Research."

Self-awareness and self-assessment will and should produce different data over time as your nursing practice evolves and shapes itself in response to the experiences you have along your career path, and in response to your ever-emerging professional and personal identity.

Who Are You?

In addition to being unique and complex, who you are is certainly more than the job you do. As was stated earlier, your job is a small segment of the work you do, which in turn reflects your mission or purpose in life, rooted in the values you believe, and the vision you have for how it all fits together. As you continuously develop and refine the answers to this question, you solidify what is permanently yours, thereby strengthening yourself to withstand shifts in marketplace needs with the capacity to find new places to "plant" yourself whenever you want or need to.

To begin, ask yourself whether you consider your nursing practice a job or a career. Which of the following definitions most closely resembles how you are currently working, or at least what you believe about your work as a nurse? A *job* belongs to someone else, is given to you for a period of time, not necessarily determined by you, and can be modified at the will of the employer, not always with your input or permission. A *career* is a proactive experience of choice based on your life purpose (your mission), guided by your vision, and grounded in your values. It is expressed in a series of (often) temporary work experiences called jobs.

Those of you who believe you have jobs rather than careers are more likely to get derailed by the hurricane-force winds of change currently blowing through the healthcare industry. But those of you who believe you have careers will instead discover and inhabit the eye of the storm, still moving with the direction of change but traveling with more inner stability and career security. In some ways, whether you call your nursing practice a job or a career may matter less in the long run than how you think about it or act in it. After all, a career does not have to be pursued full-time for a lifetime without interruption for other pursuits, such as family and friends. What is more important is that you develop a self-employed attitude about it, leading to proactive rather than passive thoughts and actions, ensuring satisfying and productive work no matter how the healthcare system restructures itself.

While there are many ways to answer the question, "Who are you?," the ones that will be explored here are: (1) what your mission, or purpose in nursing, is; (2) what your values and needs are; and (3) what your vision is for how your work as a nurse should look.

Your Mission

An ad that once ran for a major New York City Medical Center read as follows: "Providing Compassionate Quality Healthcare Isn't Our Job . . . . It's Our Mission." Committing yourself to the definition and development of your own mission statement moves you closer to the kind of productive and satisfying work that has the potential to fulfill you rather than burn you out. This will stabilize you during this Healthcare Revolution.

Developing Your Mission

A mission is the evolving expression of what you believe your purpose in life to be. It is based on innate as well as learned abilities. It includes preferences for life activities (of which work is a part) that are rooted in your value system and aligned with your vision. In her book, *The Path*, Laurie Beth Jones describes a mission statement as a "written-down reason for being; key to finding your path in life and to identifying the mission you choose to follow; having a clearly articulated mission statement gives one a template of purpose that can be used to initiate, evaluate, and refine all of one's activities."

It is this "template of purpose" that contributes to the foundation of your inner stability and career security. It can become the basis of your career path, especially if you engage in the process of "initiating, evaluating, and refining activities" by conducting the kind of semiannual self-review suggested here. This is a solid way to ground yourself as you move forward while change whirls around you. Ways of strengthening the data you get from this kind of self-review include networking with peers and colleagues for support and feedback, seeking out mentors, engaging in personal development work such as psychotherapy, and attending personal development seminars.

Jones says that finding one's mission, and then fulfilling it, is "perhaps the most vital activity in which a person can engage." This is echoed by Steven Covey, author of *The Seven Habits of Highly Effective People* and *Putting First Things First*. Covey says that a mission statement is a "philosophy or creed which focuses on what you want to be (character) and do (contributions and achievements) and on the values (principles) upon which being and doing is based." It is a "written standard, a personal constitution, and like the United States Constitution, based on the self-evident truths of the Declaration of Independence; it is fundamentally changeless, defended and supported, pledged allegiance to, and enables people to ride through such major traumas as war; it empowers individuals with tireless strength in the midst of change."

Writing Your Mission Statement

A mission statement is not something you write overnight or in one sitting. Rather, it evolves over time. According to Covey, it takes "deep introspection, careful analysis, and thoughtful expression," as you reflect on where you've been and how it has affected you, where you want to go, and what you want your life to be about. Because it is a solid expression of your values and vision, it should not be written in isolation from them.

Jones describes the elements of a mission statement as:

- No longer than a single sentence
- Easily understood by a 12-year-old
- Able to be recited automatically, by memory
- Perfectly suited to you

Both the Covey and Jones books describe excellent processes and exercises that can result in the development of a clear and powerful mission statement, and have been referred to you for further reading (see the appendix).

The following exercise, adapted from *The Path*, can be used as a way to get started on this important aspect of your career development. This exercise is the culmination of introspective explorations that get you in touch with the essence of who you are. Try out part of it here as a way to determine how far along in the process you might already be:

There are three steps to creating your mission statement.

> **Step 1** = What you do, expressed in three action verbs

Step 2 = What you stand for; the principles, causes you would defend to the death; your core value or values

Step 3 = Whom you want to help; whom you really want to serve, be around, inspire, learn from, impact, and make a difference for.

Step 1

Select three words from the list of action verbs below that most excite you, shed light on who you are, describe what you most like to spend your time doing. (This is a partial list of what is more complete in *The Path*).

facilitate	foster	alleviate	prepare	realize
communicate	improve	involve	motivate	educate
support	empower	sustain	enhance	organize

Write the three words representing what you here: _____ _____ _____

Step 2

Write a word or key phrase that describes your core value or values, the principle or principles you would defend to the death, such as *joy* or *service* or *justice* or *independence*. For additional value words, consult the list of values later in this chapter.

Write what you stand for here: _____

Step 3

Describe who you want to help. The more specific, the better. Consider the kind of healthcare client, the patient population or nursing specialty, the age group, etcetera.

Write whom you help here: _____

_____

Creating Your Mission Statement

Combine the words from Steps 1–3 to form your mission statement. Fill in the blanks.

My mission is to:

_____, _____, and _____

(your three verbs from Step 1: What you do)

_____

(your core value or values from Step 2: What you stand for)

to, for, among, in, or with:

_____

(the group or cause that most moves or excites you from Step 3: Whom you help)

Sample Mission Statement: Betsy

Betsy, a staff nurse in the ob-gyn department of a community hospital wrote the following mission statement when she learned her position in the labor and delivery unit had been eliminated:

My mission is to <u>nurture, educate, and facilitate</u>   <u>health and well-being</u> in
                              (what she does)   *(what she stands for)*

<u>traditional as well as nontraditional families, including single mothers.</u>
                              (whom she helps)

Writing it helped Betsy to recognize that the employer could take away only her job, not her work, not her career, and certainly not her mission. It helped her to focus on what she wanted her next work experience to be and what employer might be most interested in what she had to offer.

Additional examples of mission statements representative of the nurse's work include:

<u>Facilitate, teach, and encourage</u> the <u>mental and emotional health</u> of <u>inner-city school children.</u>

<u>Inspire, recognize, and promote</u> <u>healing</u> in <u>grieving adults.</u>

<u>Communicate, demonstrate, and encourage</u> <u>computer literacy</u> among <u>healthcare professionals.</u>

<u>Model, nurture, and facilitate</u> <u>empowerment</u> in <u>single mothers.</u>

<u>Inspire, improve, and sustain</u> <u>self-care and independence</u> in <u>"the oldest old" (people over 85).</u>

<u>Develop, prepare, and circulate</u> <u>diabetic teaching materials</u> for <u>newly diagnosed children.</u>

Your Values and Needs

Values are the beliefs that ground your decisions and activities in the work world and in your personal life as well. They are the expression of deeply held beliefs about how you like things to be and what you prefer to experience. Values are often based on and influenced by such psychological needs as to be with people, to be independent, to be useful, to experience stability, to influence, to serve, etcetera, as articulated in Step Two of your mission statement.

Values shape your interests and contribute to the skills you choose to learn and the accomplishments you achieve. They are the basis for the personal interests you pursue and the career paths you select, so understanding your values and needs is an essential component of the question, "Who Are You?" It is a place to start when you want to determine your next career move, or when you need to understand why you are not satisfied with your current work experience.

Take Orinthia, for example, who currently works in the newborn nursery of a community hospital. She has worked in this hospital for four years and this is her third assignment in the obstetrical department, where nurses rotate for six-month periods to each clinical area, including the ambulatory care clinics. She is experiencing the same kind of boredom and restlessness that she remembers having twice before; once when she worked on the postpartum unit, and before that, when she worked in the prenatal clinic. The one time during this current rotation that she remembered feeling genuinely interested in her work was when it was decided that infants experiencing mild respiratory distress would no longer be transferred out to the neonatal intensive care unit (NICU) of a major medical center for treatment. Instead, the nurses in the newborn nursery would be taught the skills needed to care for these infants. She learned the assessment and technical skills quickly, and in fact became a resource to two of her Nurse Colleagues, Barbara and Joan, who found these critical care tasks overwhelming. When these nurses investigated what values and needs may be represented by their preferences for work assignments, it became clear that there were some striking differences among them. Orinthia identified the following needs and values:

Challenge—work that is mentally stimulating

Detail work—performance of tasks requiring accurate focus and attention

Fast pace—meet demanding expectations within time deadlines

Excitement—work characterized by frequent novelty and drama

Variety—frequent change in job responsibilities

Barbara and Joan, the nurses who felt overwhelmed with this new assignment, identified the following values and needs:

Predictability—satisfaction with routine, repetitious tasks

Expertness—being good at something

Mastery—acquired proficiency and expertise in tasks

Connection—giving and receiving caring, support, and warmth

While all three nurses loved working with mothers and babies, Orinthia preferred caring for the sicker infants while her peers did not. In addition, Orinthia realized that practically none of the work preferences that were representative of her values and needs were typically experienced during her past rotations to the postpartum unit or the prenatal clinic, and were only present in this current rotation to the nursery when she was assigned to care for these sick infants. During those times, she felt challenged by the potential unpredictability of the sick infant's health status and the fast-paced work requiring attention to detail that was missing for her in the routine care of well babies, exactly what her peers enjoyed.

These nurses were able to request work assignments that provided more work satisfaction and less stress from feeling bored or overwhelmed because they clarified how their values and needs influenced their work preferences. Orinthia was assigned to care for the infants with respiratory distress whenever possible, while the other nurses performed the tasks more routinely associated with the nursery and more aligned with their values and preferences, including well-baby care, teaching, and emotional support of new parents. Eventually, Orinthia went to work in the obstetrical department of hospital that didn't require rotation through all of its subspecialties, and was permanently assigned to the NICU, where the fast pace suited her perfectly and was aligned with her mission to "Support, facilitate, or strengthen connection in the mother-baby bond of critically ill newborns."

To explore and clarify your needs and values as they relate to your work preferences, to your mission, and to your vision, and to the larger question of "Who Are You?," reflect on the list of values and needs in the exercise on the following pages (adapted from *The Lifetime Career Manager: New Strategies for a New Era*, by James C. Cabrera and Charles F. Albrecht). These needs and values are common to the nursing experience.

SELF-ASSESSMENT EXERCISE: YOUR NEEDS AND VALUES

Rank the following needs and values and their descriptions according to the following scale:

1 = Always necessary. Impossible or very hard to work or live without

2 = Often necessary. Could work or live without it, if necessary, or temporarily, but wouldn't want to, would miss it a lot

3 = Sometimes necessary. Would prefer to have it, but could manage fairly well if it wasn't there

4 = Rarely or never necessary. Could easily work or live without it; don't think about it much

Score	Value	Description
_____	Achievement	Attain and maintain a sense of accomplishment and mastery
_____	Aesthetics	Work in a setting that values the beauty of things and ideas
_____	Affection	Express and receive warmth and caring
_____	Authenticity	Be genuinely yourself
_____	Balance	Achieve satisfactory proportion between work and personal life
_____	Career advancement	Experience opportunities for vertical mobility (promotion), as well as horizontal mobility (transfer) within the workplace
_____	Challenge	Experience work as mentally stimulating
_____	Competition	Achieve mastery by competing with others or by challenging yourself
_____	Creativity	Express imagination and ingenuity in work
_____	Detail work	Perform tasks requiring accurate focus and detail
_____	Efficient organization	Work in an organization that runs effectively with minimal bureaucracy

Score	Value	Description
_____	Excitement	Experience adventure, frequent novelty and drama
_____	Expertness	Feeling skilled, being good at something
_____	Emotional resilience	Ability to mediate and process personal feelings and bounce back from interpersonal difficulties
_____	Fast pace	Meet demanding expectations within time deadlines
_____	Family	Experience contented personal relationships or living situation
_____	Friendship	Develop social and personal relationships with peers and colleagues
_____	Health	Pursue physical, mental, and emotional well-being
_____	Helping others	Contribute to or assist others in need
_____	Independence	Control the type of work you do, including schedule
_____	Integrity	Work ethically and honestly
_____	Knowledge	Learn and use specific information
_____	Leadership	Influence, authorize, or direct others to achieve results
_____	Location	Live in a convenient geographical location in a suitable community
_____	Management	Achieve work goals as a result of the efforts of others
_____	Money	Reap significant financial rewards
_____	Meaningful work	Perform work that has purpose, relevance

Score	Value	Description
_____	Personal growth	Develop and grow into your potential
_____	Pleasure	Experience enjoyment, fun, satisfaction
_____	Physical health	Express vitality and well being
_____	Positive atmosphere	Work in a pleasing, supportive, harmonious setting
_____	Power	Control the resources at work
_____	Recognition	Receive credit and appreciation for work well done; be known or well-known; be praised
_____	Security	Work without fear of unemployment, have stable future
_____	Service	Contribute to the well-being, welfare, or satisfaction of another
_____	Spirituality	Express meaning of life or religious beliefs
_____	Status	Attain a position of recognized importance
_____	Variety and change	Perform tasks of great variety
_____	Wisdom	Develop insight and understanding
_____	Work with others	Belong to a satisfying work group or team

Interpreting Your Score

In reviewing this self-assessment, notice how many 1's and 2's you have and whether your work or personal life is set up to allow their expression. The 1's and 2's relate to values and needs that should not be compromised—at least not for too long, because it can lead to personal and interpersonal conflict, stress, and eventually to burnout.

The 3's and 4's are places where you can allow yourself more leeway in trying to realign with the reality of the situation.

To the degree that your values are blocked from expression in either or both places, you may be living out of balance and harmony with who you are. While it is unrealistic to expect the workplace to match all of your values and needs, a preponderance of them needs to be met for work satisfaction and productivity to be present. A perfect prescription for stress is a value system that is very misaligned with the work you are doing. Rather than overlook or minimize the importance of this on your personal well-being and career satisfaction, if you do discover a misalignment, consider the following options:

Compensate for Your Unmet Values

Compensate for what is missing by identifying other places for their expression. For example, if Personal Growth is a "1" and you are not experiencing this at work, consider where else in your life this can be accommodated. Consider taking courses or enrolling in seminars, joining a support group, or engaging in the personal inquiry process through psychotherapy.

Negotiate for Your Values

Negotiate for the value or need that is not being fulfilled. For example, if you scored a 1 or 2 for recognition, and it is in short supply where you work, try asking for feedback more often or consider participating in a work activity that might provide some consistent appreciation for a job well done, perhaps committee work.

Realign Your Values

This does not mean compromise or giving up what keeps you rooted to the essence of who you are. To realign your values means to evaluate what your current job can realistically provide and to see if you can modify your expectations accordingly. This might be possible if you know that the job you have is temporary, or if you design your personal life so that there are ample opportunities for the expression of the needs or values blocked at work.

For example, if you scored a 1 or 2 for "Power" (controlling resources at work) and this is not within your current job responsibilities, try to relate to what *is* there, not what you wish could be, learning to let go of what you can't control. This could be a growth experience as you learn to accommodate yourself to the reality of your experience rather than fighting to change the unchangeable.

However, selecting this option requires paying very careful attention to the line between flexibility and total compromise of values and needs. Many acute care nurses, and nurses in general, are facing this dilemma when it comes to the higher volume of patients requiring care in shorter periods of time so that hospital revenues are maintained during these times of managed care. The phrase *do more with less* is such an affront to the nursing value system of safe, ethical patient care that each situation in which you find yourself confronted with this experience requires a careful examination of what can be compromised and what cannot. In reality, there are times when it *is* possible to do more, faster, and with fewer people, and there are also times when it is not. The guiding barometer and final arbiter for this will be you, as you develop self-awareness about your values and needs and determine how they are matched with your current place of employment.

Another situation that may require some values realignment is the application of a business philosophy and strategies to the value of caring for people in the healthcare industry. You could argue that there is an inherent incompatibility between these two concepts and that mixing them creates unethical and potentially unsafe scenarios. While it is true that the ruthless application of a bottom-line business mentality can indeed compromise patient safety, it is just as hard to argue against how the possibility of more effective health care delivery systems could finally emerge from the chaos of nonsystems in healthcare.

The best way of viewing these two concepts is to eliminate the polarization of black and white thinking and find some gray in it, some middle ground where each might exist side by side. This kind of reframing and revisioning of thought and perception is essential during these times of paradox and permanent transition.

Honor and Stand Up for Your Values

Decide whether a career move, and perhaps a new career path, is necessary because your values are either too compromised, or just cannot be met where you are. If control of resources is essential to you and realigning your expectations is not possible, ask yourself why you're working in a place that can't meet these needs. If your answer has more to do with salary and employment benefits than your overall career goals, you might benefit from prioritizing your needs and values, perhaps with a mentor or coach who can provide objective feedback and guidance so that you can keep your career progress on track. If you believe that the latest changes in your workplace have made it impossible to provide safe, effective care, you would be better off working where your values and needs about patient care delivery could more easily be met. So would your employer, and so would the patients you cares for.

Another way to stand up for what you believe is to help fight for what you are not able to influence by yourself. For example, supporting the successful media campaign of the New York State Nurses Association that "Every Patient Deserves a Nurse" is a way to have your values and beliefs expressed. Joining the American Nurses Association and participating directly through committee work or indirectly though membership dues is another way to honor and stand up for your nursing practice values.

Developing Your Vision

Robert Kennedy said "Some men see things as they are and ask, 'Why?' I dream of things that could be and ask, 'Why not?'" Kennedy had a vision of how the future could be, and so can you. Building your vision is the third of the three components that comprise the question, "Who Are You?" and asks you to imagine what you see yourself doing, where, and with whom, at some point in the future. It is the bridge between your mission and values, and represents the ideal place you would like to activate and experience them.

> "Today, a whole new set of career opportunities is available in nursing. The future belongs to the visionary, to those who can create new configurations to respond to new demands and who have the courage to follow their vision."
>
> —Gloria Smith, in *Managing Your Career in Nursing*

Having a vision enhances and allows for the extension, growth, and development of your mission and your values. The experience of having a vision of the future provides a stabilizing anchor in the present that can steady you through turbulent times of change while serving as a lighted beacon of hope and optimism toward which you navigate. This is especially true when you find yourself in a work situation that has changed unexpectedly and/or may no longer be aligned with your mission or your values. A vision can become a stress-management strategy because it prevents you from feeling trapped or victimized and gives you some realistic control over your destiny. You can even build a path to your vision by using your present experience as a training ground, accumulating skills and experiences that are transferable to what you envision yourself doing in the future.

For example, Clarissa values teaching and enjoys helping people feel more confident in their ability to learn complicated things. She has been working as an acute care nurse on a medical unit for four years and most enjoys teaching newly diagnosed diabetics who are feeling overwhelmed and confused about how to adapt effectively and manage their care. After her organization restructured and redesigned the nursing roles, she found herself with additional work assignments that allowed less time for teaching, even though this was still an expected part of her job. In taking stock of where she was and what she saw herself doing in the future, she realized that she wanted to combine her nursing knowledge, including the knack she had for teaching how to simplify complicated things, with her interest in computers. She heard about the new role of the nurse informatics specialist and began to imagine herself doing that. What she would be doing and where was vague, but the more she imagined it and allowed for its possibility, the more motivated she felt about exploring what it would take to make it happen.

When she heard that the hospital was offering computer classes, she jumped at the chance to enroll. She also volunteered to work on a teaching task force that was investigating how to use computers for the teaching and learning needs of the nursing staff. Her dissatisfaction with her newly redesigned job was easier to tolerate because she used every opportunity she could to add to the skills she believed were transferable to her future vision. She volunteered to assist in the development of standardized teaching plans to make the teaching role of busy or novice nurses easier. She found resources for and developed teaching kits with handouts that simplified concepts and saved time. And she pored over the want ads to learn what the qualifications were for nurse informatics specialist, what kind of organizations used them. She read about this role, attended seminars about it, and eventually entered a graduate nursing program that prepared nurses for it. Clarissa used her vision to encourage her forward movement, strengthen her mission and values, and make creative use of an otherwise unacceptable present situation.

Creating a vision relies mostly on the thinking style of the right brain, where thought occurs in mental impressions, fleeting images, and intuitive hunches. It is the twin partner to the logical processing and sequential reasoning of the left brain. Using both abilities results in a more complete picture of your career hopes and dreams, plans, and goals. While thinking about the future with your left brain results in goals, tasks, and checklists, thinking about the future with your right brain becomes a strategy to encourage and even accelerate forward momentum towards your hopes and dreams so that the difficulties often inherent in the fulfillment of your mission and values do not overwhelm or discourage you.

Right-brain thought is rich with the information and also the support needed to move into the future, but because rational reasoning is favored as the dominant thinking style of the scientifically based western world, the right brain receives less training and validation. Creative right brain activities are not always understood or encouraged. As a child, you may remember daydreaming (an essential function of creativity and vision building) and being told by a parent or teacher that you were not paying attention. Or perhaps you were told not to let your imagination run away with you as you wrote a story or spoke to an imaginary playmate. These normal, creative, and eminently useful right-brain thinking processes can be recaptured by devoting a little time and effort to relearning and remembering them, and by suspending judgment and criticism of the process as well as the results.

Tips and Guidelines for the Development of Your Vision

Write It Down

Write down your vision and recall it frequently. Then say it aloud, to yourself at first, always using present-tense vocabulary. Writing it down provides a kind of contract with yourself, and speaking about it in the present tense acts as a feedback loop to strengthen it and your resolve when the going gets tough. Share it with people who encourage and believe in you. Hearing yourself talk about it out loud reinforces the reality of it and helps move it from the possible to the probable, and eventually into the actual.

Take Your Vision Outside Your Comfort Zone

Allow your vision to stretch you beyond your comfort zone without being unrealistic or overly ambitious, as Marcia Perkins-Reed advocates in her book, *Thriving in Transition*. She writes, "It should challenge us to reach further than we have before. If we do this at each of our transitional junctures, we will be constantly growing into greater possibilities. So if we think we can easily earn $25,000 in our next position, a minimum salary of $27,500 or $30,000 should appear in our vision statement. While we don't want to push ourselves relentlessly, ever striving towards elusive new goals that we don't believe will bring us success, we do want to expand our vision into the highest and best situation we can imagine knowing that what we attract may be even better than that!"

Don't Let Stress Be an Obstacle

Tolerate the stress and tension that naturally exists between your future vision and your present reality. Robert Fritz in *The Path of Least Resistance* describes this as essential to the creative process that will eventually manifest your vision. He suggests that it is necessary to hold in your mind the simultaneous experiences of how you want your life to be and how your life actually is now. The gap between these two experiences will narrow in favor of the path that offers the least resistance. To tolerate the tension between your present reality and your future vision means to develop plans and utilize stress management strategies that support your movement toward your vision, rather than to collapse your vision into your present reality because the tension is too difficult to tolerate.

Be Patient

Don't expect your vision to occur immediately or be crystal clear in its guidance. Clarity will emerge over time as the experiences you have along the way shape and enhance the vision further. It may take a while to arrive at your vision, as you review and revise it over the time it takes to get there. In truth, for those who learn to use this kind of visionary guidance, arrival is a short-lived experience on the way to a continually evolving future always just tantalizingly out of reach. Your vision, like your life, is an ever-unfolding process, a journey over time, not necessarily a destination. Learning to relish the experience of getting there as much as the arrival is an excellent way to approach life in permanent transition and constant change that is common today. This does not mean that goals are never achieved, but rather that where you have arrived is a step to what is always next, what is always being reviewed and revised.

Stay Focused on the Future

Reflect frequently on the question, "Where do you see yourself in the future? Doing what, with whom?" Consider starting a journal to capture and track the progressive development of your vision, using it as encouragement and motivation. Or carry a small notebook with you to capture fleeting thoughts or images related to your vision in your spare time. Often, when you turn your attention away from something you've been pondering, clarity emerges unexpectedly and spontaneously.

A Vision Exercise

Everyone has the capacity to visualize. The more you practice this ability, the stronger it will become. In some ways, visualizing is just another way of thinking which you do more often than you realize. To demonstrate this, bring to mind your living room. Take about 15 seconds to recall the room and its contents, including any colors, associated sounds, or even aromas or physical sensations.

Most likely, you thought about your living room not in words but in images, or formed mental impressions of where the furnishings and objects of your living room were. Perhaps you even thought about some associated sensory experiences like aromas or sounds. It would be highly unusual for you to have conjured up words to describe your living room. Instead, you most likely imagined it, visualized it, and saw it on the movie screen of your mind. In the same way, you can create images of your future and thereby build your vision. Start by reflecting on and answering the questions below.

Begin by sitting quietly in a comfortable place in which you won't be interrupted for at least 30 minutes.

Prepare yourself by performing a breathing or relaxation exercise that quiets your mind, allows you to turn inward, and creates a receptive attitude within you. See the appendix for additional information on both relaxation exercises and vision building.

Reflect on the following questions and imagine the answers in images rather than thinking about them in words: "Where do you see yourself? Doing what, with whom? In one year? In five years? In 10 years? Or at some other time in the future?" Keep the emphasis on seeing and imagining yourself and what is going on around you, allowing images and impressions to be filled in. Avoid developing a mental list of what you may know you need to do, the plans and goals you may already have or know you need to develop. Remember, you want to stimulate right-brain creative processes rather than left-brain problem solving.

When you have reflected, imagined, and envisioned the answers that emerged from the exercise above, and perhaps pondered them over time, use what you have discovered to create your vision statement here:

_____

_____

_____

_____

_____

What Do You Have to Offer?

Part of knowing what you have to offer as a nurse is being clear about what you are good at—what you prefer to spend the majority of your time doing. This may be confusing because there are so many options and opportunities from which to choose. An approach that provides some clarity is to understand how the nursing role contains basic work skills or activities that are blended with core nursing competencies. At best, however, even this approach can provide only general guidelines because

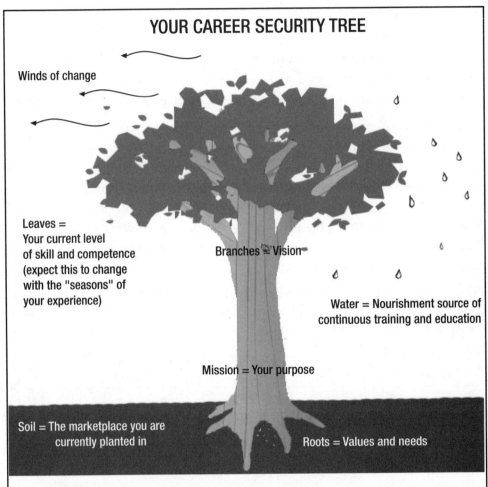

YOUR CAREER SECURITY TREE

Winds of change

Leaves =
Your current level
of skill and competence
(expect this to change
with the "seasons" of
your experience)

Branches = Vision

Water = Nourishment source of
continuous training and education

Mission = Your purpose

Soil = The marketplace you are
currently planted in

Roots = Values and needs

The Career Security Tree captures and summarizes a schematic answer to the questions of "Who are you?" and "What do you have to offer?" to remind you that (1) who you are has more ever-growing permanence than your temporary job, (2) you can transplant who you are into the "soil" of new employment territory, and (3) you can grow, especially when the winds of change blow.

Your personal security tree must be firmly rooted, with its branches going with the flow, so that they can not be blown away by change.

nursing roles resist strict categorization. They are extremely fluid, very influenced by the unique patient care needs of a particular setting, and to some degree, open to the personal interpretation of the nurse performing the role (or perhaps, the nurse manager who may have created the role). Nursing roles are also responsive to marketplace trends and changes, including the reengineering of hospitals systems with its resulting redesign of nursing job descriptions. Hence, a nurse manager in one setting might work very differently from a nurse manager in another setting. Likewise, the job description for the role of the medical-surgical staff nurse will look quite different after a hospital has reengineered its patient care delivery system. This creative interpretation is what makes nursing practice so interesting, versatile, and creative.

Blending the Basic Work Activities with Core Nursing Competencies

There are three general categories of basic work activities performed by nurses: (1) people skills, (2) data and information skills, and (3) concept and idea skills. These skills exist in almost all the work you do, and are blended into the core nursing competencies of clinical, managerial, educational, interpersonal, and technical expertise. Some authorities identify the additional competencies of political, commercial, and governance. Combining these nursing competencies with basic work skills creates a nursing role. Examples are listed in the box on the next page.

Core Nursing Competencies

Below are generalized overviews of the most common core competencies in nursing. Since these competencies are rarely performed in isolation from one another, the overlap in describing them is reflective of the creative complexity of nursing practice.

Clinical Competencies

These competencies describe the direct relationship a nurse has with a patient. It involves using specific technical skills within the nursing process steps of assessment, planning, intervention, and evaluation, for the purpose of influencing, supporting, or sustaining a patient's particular physical or emotional needs. Clinical competencies

BASIC WORK SKILLS

People Skills	Data and Information Skills	Concept and Idea Skills
counseling	systematizing	creating
motivating	using logic	translating
advocating	classifying information	visualizing
empathizing	analyzing facts	conceptualizing
coaching	compiling information	synthesizing
persuading	summarizing	inventing
facilitating	working with numbers	designing
delegating	testing hypothesis	symbolizing
training	allocating resources	acting
teaching	keeping records	innovating
listening	tabulating	extrapolating
advising	budgeting	demonstrating
interviewing	keeping inventories	communicating
resolving conflicts	using logic	evaluating
collaborating	editing	presenting
providing	mediating	reviewing
performing	negotiating	assisting
assessing	informing	developing
appreciating	regulating	interpreting
intervening	assigning	imagining
accomplishing	appreciating	affecting
alleviating	combining	affirming
defending	directing	confirming
enhancing	devising	empowering
healing	gathering	encouraging
improving	generating	fostering
nurturing	manifesting	illuminating
safeguarding	revising	involving
supporting	planning	persuading
sustaining	progressing	praising
touching	validating	translating

are used by all nurses who provide direct care to patients. All other nursing competencies (described below) are inextricably woven together with these clinical competencies. Likewise, many of the work abilities related to people, data and information, and concept and idea skills are often represented in clinical nursing competencies, expressed in a variety of clinical nursing roles. Examples of these clinical competencies, typically performed in the clinical role of the medical surgical nurse at the novice or expert level, might include:

- Caring for postoperative patients
- Inserting IV lines
- Counseling families of dying patients
- Calculating medications
- Planning for discharge
- Teaching self-care to patients
- Interpreting data from monitor readouts
- Mentoring new nurses

Interpersonal Competencies

These competencies involve communicating with and relating to others. They often reflect —but are not limited to—the basic activities involved in people skills and concept and idea skills. Since clinical competencies cannot exist without interpersonal competencies, some of the examples from above could just as easily be used here, such as teaching self-care to patients, mentoring new nurses, and counseling families of dying patients. Additional examples might include:

- Facilitating medication groups
- Empathizing with an anxious patient
- Collaborating with physicians
- Actively listening to a family members concern
- Advocating for patients rights
- Resolving conflicts between home health aides

Managerial Competencies

These competencies primarily involve planning, organizing, directing, and controlling system resources as well as the people in them. Data and information skills are often correlated with managerial competencies. General managerial competencies are part of the role of the direct care nurse providing direct patient care, as well as the Nurse Manager who oversees it. Examples include:

- Supervising nursing staff
- Conducting studies of sick time utilization
- Writing annual performance evaluations
- Writing handbooks for patient care technicians
- Using computers to develop budgets
- Designing new patient care delivery system
- Coordinating patient care activities
- Delegating responsibilities to others

Educational Competencies

These competencies primarily involve communicating concepts and ideas to others by means of explaining, teaching, and coaching. Once again, educational competencies are closely related to all the other nursing competencies, including, of course, interpersonal competencies. Examples include:

- Teaching CPR to new mothers
- Teaching glucometer use to diabetic patient
- Designing nursing school curriculum
- Creating orientation programs
- Mentoring new graduates
- Presenting online learning programs

Technical Competencies

These competencies involve the use of equipment and machinery, often complex and computerized, in correlation with other nursing competencies. Technical competencies rely heavily on the basic work abilities of data and information skills, and cut across all nursing roles, in one way or another. High-tech and low-tech examples include:

EXAMPLES OF NURSING ROLES CORRELATED WITH CORE COMPETENCIES

Clinical Competencies

All nurses involved in direct patient care, and:

Adult nurse practitioner

Psychiatric direct care nurse specialist

Community health nurse

Telephone triage nurse

Managerial Competencies

All nurses involved in direct patient care, and:

Nurse manager in a cardiac care center

Vice president, nursing and patient care services

Nurse researcher

Case manager

Educational Competencies

All nurses involved in direct patient care, and:

Staff development specialist

Professor, college of nursing

Community health educator

Childbirth educator

Interpersonal Competencies

All nurses involved in direct patient care, and:

Parish nurse

Bereavement counselor

Addictions and substance abuse specialist

Nurse psychotherapist

Technical Competencies

All nurses involved in direct patient care, and:

Nurse informatics specialist

Critical care nurse

High tech home care nurse

Sales representative for high tech company

- Regulating ventilators
- Presenting online learning programs
- Taking blood pressures
- Hemodynamic monitoring
- Obtaining blood samples from central IV lines
- Using computers to input lab data
- Performing wound care
- Using computers to develop budgets

The Colors of Your Nursing Palette

Just like the primary colors of red, yellow, and blue form the basis of a vast color palate, so does the blending of these basic work skills with the core nursing competencies determine the "color" of your nursing practice palate. Nurses who prefer people skills make excellent direct care nurses at the novice or expert level as long as they also develop the work skills and nursing competencies that accompany the role as expected by their current employer. These often vary from workplace to workplace and might include a higher or lower proportion of data and information skills or concept and idea skills. Likewise, nurses with a high preference for data and information skills make good nurse managers, and generally speaking, nurses with a high preference for concept and idea skills make good nurse educators.

These categories of basic work skills and core nursing competencies are best conceptualized as potential career pathways to the great number of clinical, administrative, educational, research, and consultation options in your nursing career.

These include, for example: Adult nurse practitioner, occupational health nurse, nurse entrepreneur, medical-surgical staff nurse, nurse researcher, staff development specialist, infection control nurse, case manager, and so on.

Chapter 8, "Marketplace Research," will elaborate on these roles and discuss the healthcare environments in which they can be found. See Appendix A for sources that will provide a detailed description of many nursing roles, including career profiles.

> ## YOUR NURSING ROLE IS A BLENDING OF:
>
> *Basic work skills*   +   *Core nursing competencies*   =   *Your nursing role*
>
> | | | |
> |---|---|---|
> | May include several categories of skills, with one or more in dominant use | May include more than one competency, with one or more being used primarily | direct care nurse, or nurse manager, or staff development specialist, et cetera |

The Effect of Healthcare Restructuring on Nursing Roles

The redesign of nursing job descriptions occurring as a result of healthcare restructuring is changing how your work skills and core nursing competencies are blended. This can sometimes lead to role conflict, confusion, and often to increased levels of stress. Let's say you're a staff nurse in an acute care hospital that has restructured its services. Suddenly, you may find yourself with a smaller percentage of the people skills and clinical competencies you prefer and have always done, while the patient care technician you now supervise moves closer to providing the direct patient care you once did. In your redesigned role, you may be expected to spend a larger portion of your time in the managerial competencies of supervising, planning, and delegating than you would prefer. One solution to this conflict may lie within you: You can make an effort to track where along the Continuum of Care the kind of work that you prefer now exists (see chapter 8, "Marketplace Research"). Another way you could resolve this conflict is by adapting to the newly redesigned role, seeing it as a challenge with new skills to learn. This may not be the best approach for all nurses, but it can be an interesting option for many.

Levels of Nursing Proficiency

Another factor to consider in determining what you have to offer is the status or progression of your nursing career path, expressed by your level of proficiency. Pat Benner's classic and oft-quoted work, *From Novice to Expert*, is useful in making this determination, and then ultimately helpful in deciding what you have to offer potential employers as well as what the next step in your career path might be. Benner describes the five possible stages each role has as novice, advanced beginner, competent, proficient, and expert.

A *novice* has no experience in the role to be performed; for example, the newly graduated nurse or nurse practitioner. The *advanced beginner* has limited, recurring experience; for example, a new B.S.N. graduate with nine months experience on a medical-surgical unit. The level called *competent* describes a nurse who has at least two years of experience performing the same role. At the level Benner calls *proficient*, the nurse can practice in situations requiring greater speed and flexibility, generally thought to occur after performing the role for three to five years. Nurses practicing at the *expert* level have achieved an intuitive and immediate level of mastery in complex situations thought to occur after a period of five or more years of experience in the same role.

Each time you move between the generic roles of clinician, manager, or educator, there may be a need to move through these proficiency levels again. You will bring to your new role what you've learned along the way in the form of transferable skills, abilities, and experiences. While this may help you move up the hierarchy in your new role, the very act of practicing in a new role can lead to some insecurity. You might feel uncomfortable unless you come to understand the need to progress along this learning curve through to the next proficiency level.

Take Karen, for example. An ANCC board-certified (at the generalist level) medical surgical staff nurse with 10 years of experience in a variety of inpatient and ambulatory settings, including critical care, Karen is practicing at the expert level according to Benner's model. Upon graduation from the adult nurse practitioner program that she has been attending for the last two years, she could be considered a novice in that role and will need to give herself time to progress again through the levels of nursing practice proficiency. A lack of tolerance for this necessary transition can result in a loss of confidence that might prevent Karen from seeking employment as a nurse practitioner.

Technological Competence Spans All Nursing Roles

A fourth category of basic skills that spans across all nursing roles is technological proficiency. No industry, especially healthcare, is immune from the march of the technological drummer. While there are some nursing practice options that will require less technological proficiency, you are fooling yourself if you decide to bypass this experience, hoping it will bypass you somehow. For example, some degree of technological proficiency is necessary for the direct care nurse who needs to access laboratory data, document the administration of medication, and log vital signs via bedside computer terminals. The critical care nurse performing hemodyanamic monitoring of patients on advanced life support equipment is practicing in a high-tech career option, while the ambulatory care nurse working in a medical clinic may be in a lower-tech work environment. However, not all ambulatory nursing roles involves low-tech work. Consider the technology that may be involved in some ob-gyn clinics, especially IVF departments. The nurse manager's relationship to technology may include using e-mail for interdepartmental communication and spreadsheets to develop budgets. And the nurse educator may use a computer program to develop her own overhead transparencies or create and teach online distance-learning classes. What is important is to come to terms with technology in the role you have chosen, or to seek a different role that is less technologically demanding without expecting it to be absent altogether.

The one technological skill that all nurses need no matter what their area of practice is computer skills. A computer is not a fancy typewriter. It is a way to access and process information, stay informed, and network for support.

Take the case of Ellen, for example. She's worked for three years in the neonatal intensive care unit of a major medical center. While she is satisfied with her level of competence, she is also aware of her tentativeness and periodic reluctance when assigned to care for infants on complete life support. She finds herself especially anxious about the equipment, and seems to learn it a bit slower than her peers. She dreaded the introduction of yet one more new ventilator to learn, having just begun to feel comfortable with the one introduced last year. She watches her peers exhibit much more confidence that she has. She is also aware that all aspects of care, especially teaching mothers how to care for and bond with these very fragile infants, are enormously satisfying to her. She grows to recognize that she is working with the right kind of patient, but in an environment that is too technologically challenging for her. She decides that what she has to offer could be best utilized in a home-care setting, where she could spend more time on what she is best at, namely facilitating the mother-baby bond.

Additional Product Development Strategies

Education and Training

There are two general categories of training and education to consider. The first category is the basic educational preparation that allows you entry into the nursing profession. The second category is continuing education and training that will keep your nursing competency current and marketable.

Basic Education

Presently there are three educational paths to nursing practice: (1) the four-year Bachelor of Science in Nursing (B.S.N.), preferred by most nursing leaders and considered a "first-class ticket to ride" in today's competitive job market; (2) the two-year Associate Degree (A.D.), considered more technical than theoretical in scope and believed to be a stepping stone towards the preferred BSN; and (3) the diploma, a 2–3 year experience that was more traditional prior to the 1970s and less available as a choice today.

In 1965, the American Nurses Association published a position paper advocating two levels of education and practice, with the B.S.N. to be the entry level into *professional* nursing practice, and the A.D. representing the *technical* entry level. More than 30 years later, the debate goes on without clear resolution, with the unfortunate result of confusion for the nursing community, patients, and others. Because it is generally believed that the B.S.N. degree provides a more comprehensive preparation, this is becoming a more frequent requirement of employment at both the novice and expert levels, especially during this time of healthcare restructuring and downsizing, when employers can be more selective. Until a clear mandate regarding this divisive issue emerges, you must make your own decision based on your own values, needs, and interests, as well as your knowledge of employment trends, predictions, and practices. Scanning the qualifications for the majority of nursing positions, especially in large cities, clearly demonstrates the preference for nurses prepared at the B.S.N. level. While work experience is a factor that can balance the absence of this qualification, especially if you are able to sell what you have to offer effectively in the employment interview, you may need to ask yourself if—or for how long—you want to work around this potential disadvantage. Why not liberate your energy for more creative and productive use?

If you find yourself resistant to returning to school (or in the case of someone contemplating nursing, spending four years instead of two in school), ask yourself what the best product development decision would be for You, Inc. What would a smart business person do? What would make you most competitive and most marketable? While the best decision for your present circumstances might be to start off with a two-year rather than a four-year degree, don't be lulled into complacency after obtaining it; deciding against the continuation for the B.S.N. can result in a less competitive "product" to offer.

Advanced Education

Two additional levels of education beyond the B.S.N. are the master's and the doctorate degrees. Seeking leadership roles in nursing practice, such as the nurse manager or the nurse educator, requires advanced preparation, with the doctorate often preferred for the nurse executive position or for nursing professorships in schools or colleges of nursing.

For the nurse practitioner or the nurse educator, the optimal degree is the masters in nursing. However, the future nurse manager might do quite well with an M.B.A. or similar business credential rather than a traditional nursing master's. See the appendix for more extensive discussions of these and other advanced educational options and pathways.

Continuing Education and Ongoing Training

This second general category of education refers to the lifelong pursuit of ever-improving professional competence to which every nurse must commit. This will make your product not only most attractive to potential and current employers, but also most personally satisfying.

As a nurse, you are a "knowledge worker" in a knowledge industry driven by the onward march of information and the emergence of technology at a rate that becomes dizzier and more explosive with each succeeding year. Stop learning, or get lazy about training, retraining, or crosstraining yourself, and you risk falling out of step in the work world and with those who are keeping their eye more closely on this aspect of "product development."

A training area you need to take seriously is your ability to use computers to process and access information, thereby strengthening your competitive edge as a knowledge worker. How are you preparing yourself to utilize this inescapable technology? And, while the employer is sure to provide some training and education in its use, which type of nurse do you think the employer might consider more seriously for employment: those who can discuss their experiences with computers, or those who don't have this represented either in their resume or in their dialogue with the interviewer? Which type of these nurses are you preparing to be?

Other training and educational experiences may be more closely related to your nursing sub-specialty. For example, basic cardiac life support for the medical-surgical staff nurse, advanced cardiac life support for the critical care nurse, and physical assessment skills of geriatric patients for the home care nurse.

Professional Certification

Another product development strategy that is not new but takes on new meaning in the increasingly competitive healthcare marketplace is board certification in a particular area of professional nursing practice, either at the generalist or specialist level. Certification is a way to announce and advertise your pride in achieving recognition from a professional nursing association for achieving an outstanding level of nursing practice. Healthcare organizations know the marketing power inherent in being certified as a Magnet Status Hospital from the American Nurses Credentialing Center (ANCC), a branch of the American Nurses Association. Your ANCC certification for individual nursing excellence can provide the same marketing advantage for you.

ANCC board certification at the generalist (B.S.N. required as of 1999) and specialist level (master-prepared, advanced practice nurses) is available in several areas of nursing practice, including psychiatric mental-health, medical-surgical, gerontological, pediatric, perinatal, and community health.

Certification in particular nursing specialties is also available from other professional associations. A few examples are:

Nursing Specialty	Professional Association
Critical Care Nursing (CCRN)	American Association of Critical Care Nurses
Occupational Health Nursing (COHN)	American Board for Occupational Health Nurses
Emergency Nursing (CEN) Nursing	Board of Certification for Emergency
Infection Control Nursing (CIC)	Certification Board Of Infection Control

In the next chapter, you will investigate and explore where in the marketplace you can take the nursing practice product you have.

Chapter 8

Marketplace Research

In the chapter on product development, you had an opportunity to explore two of the three questions—"Who are you?" and "What do you have to offer?"—essential to maintaining the competitive edge of You, Inc., during these times of permanent transition in healthcare. To explore the third question—"Who needs it?"—requires an understanding of what the

> "You must become aware of the richness in you and come to believe in it and know it is there . . . . Once you become aware of it and have faith in it, you will be all right."
> —Brenda Ueland

new healthcare frontier and its rapidly evolving territories look like. As the chief executive and operating officer of You, Inc., you will need to keep your eye on this fluctuating marketplace at least as often as you monitor the activities in your product development department, perhaps semiannually. All nurses desiring productive and satisfying work at the dawn of the 21st century need to be vigilant in this area.

Continuous marketplace research is an effective way to ensure that you will be able to match what you have to offer with the best and most interesting employment venue possible. Ways to conduct this research include networking with peers and colleagues in person and online, monitoring professional activities on the Internet and in the print and television media, reading books that forecast trends, receiving newsletters and publications from professional organizations such as the American Nurses Association and their affiliating state associations, and attending professional conferences and conventions.

To alert you to the critical need for this career strategy, listen to the words of Tim Porter-O'Grady, a well known and respected expert on the healthcare system and nursing practice issues: "We are watching the end of healthcare as we know it. In context, we are also seeing the end of nursing as we know it. . . . Healthcare service is changing in ways that will demand a different set of roles and characteristics for the nurse. Indeed, the opportunity to make significant change in the role of the nurse has never been stronger in the history of American nursing."

Endings herald beginnings as well. There is an emerging healthcare environment that requires profound changes in the way nurses practice. Porter-O'Grady describes these changes as "really a blessing for the nursing profession. . . . In most ways, nurses should be happy that the hospital-centric age is passing. . . . Nurses have been historically underused in hospitals. . . . The very medical model of service structures in hospitals only allowed nurses to function at a fraction of their capacity because anything beyond functional proficiency was considered the turf of the physician. Extreme medical direction and subordinacy have been the *modus operandi* for generations in hospitals throughout the country." The demise of this medical model of care and the Continuum of Care model replacing it (described below) is what will provide you with employment opportunities outside the familiar hospital walls, and within them as well, but in very different ways, and allow you to practice well beyond a fraction of your capacity.

It is practically impossible to accurately predict what the future healthcare workplace will look like, given the degree of chaotic flux occurring as the new millennium approaches. What is possible is to move You, Inc. forward based on current healthcare, societal, and employment trends and predictions, all the while making the necessary adjustments and revisions in your career path as the unfolding facts present themselves more clearly and completely.

Marketplace Research in Today's Healthcare Environment

In "The New Practice Environment," a chapter written for an anthology entitled, *Nurse Case Management in the 21st Century,* Vivien DeBack outlines the characteristics of the emerging healthcare system as described by the PEW Health Professions Commission, a nonprofit healthcare research organization. These are:

- Orientation towards health, with greater emphasis on prevention and wellness, and greater expectation for individual responsibility for healthy behaviors.

- The use of a "population perspective," in which there is new attention to risk factors affecting substantial segments of the community, including issues of access and the physical and social environment.

- Intensive use of information with reliance on information systems to provide complete, easily assimilated patient information as well as ready access to relevant information on current practice.

- Focus on the consumer, with expectation and encouragement of patient partnerships in decisions related to treatment, facilitated by the availability of complete information on outcomes and evaluated in part by patient satisfaction.

- Knowledge of treatment outcomes with emphasis on the determination of the most effective treatment under different conditions and the dissemination of this information to those involved in treatment decisions.

- Constrained resources, with a pervasive concern over increasing costs, coupled with expanded use of mechanisms to control or limit available expenditures.

- Coordination of resources, with increased integration of providers and an emphasis on teams to improve efficiency and effectiveness across all settings.

- Reconsideration of human values, with careful assessment of the balance between the expanding capability of technology and the need for humane treatment.

- Expectations of accountability, with growing scrutiny by a larger variety of payers, consumers, and regulators, coupled with more formally defined performance expectations.

- Growing interdependence, with further integration of domestic issues of health, education, and public safety combined with a growing awareness of the importance of healthcare in a global context.

The following words summarize *The PEW Commissions Report*, highlighting the trends and predictions relevant to nursing employment, the kind of nursing practice that can be expected, and what is required for skills building and acquisition.

- Prevention, healthy behaviors, wellness
- Information technologies, information systems
- Consumer focus, including patient satisfaction
- Treatment outcomes, treatment decisions
- Constrained resources, control mechanisms, limited expenditures
- Improved efficiency, integrated teams
- Human values, humane treatment
- Accountability, scrutiny by payers, regulators
- Global context

Cultural and Societal Trends and Predictions

There are profound changes occurring at every level of society, resulting in individual, organizational, and global transformations. These include:

- A shift from the Industrial Age of manufacturing to the Information Age where the currency is knowledge and information
- A focus on primary prevention, wellness, and holistic healthcare practices
- Patients who are smarter consumers and want partnership in their relationships with all healthcare providers
- A new model of work, with shorter-term employment in more than one industry, increase in flexible work schedules, and more work being done from home
- Increasing numbers of women, ethnic minorities, and workers between the ages of 45 and 54. The Bureau of Labor Statistics predicts that by the year

2000, women will make up 47 percent of the workforce, and 61 percent of all women will be working.

• A growing awareness that age is a state of mind, especially as the United States population ages. By the year 2030, 20 percent of the people will be over age 65, with the fastest growing segment being those over age 80. Most of the elderly will be living in the community, alone, with aging spouses, or with their children or other relatives.

How and where nurses will be working will emerge gradually as these trends and predictions become realities, accompanied by a new model of preventative healthcare that will replace the illness-focused nonsystem prevalent today. The emerging model of healthcare involves a consumer-oriented, wellness-focused, economically feasible system of primary care. It will offer services along a continuum, ranging from prevention through acute to postacute care, delivered where people reside or work, including their homes, communities, schools, places of employment, and houses of worship.

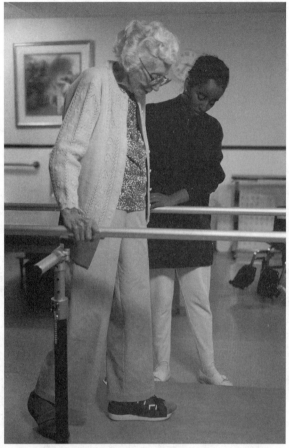

By the year 2030, 20 percent of the people will be over age 65, with the fastest growing segment being those over age 80. This is a major market for all nurses to consider.

Sheila A. Ryan, in "Academia's Involvement in Healthcare's Redesign," another chapter from the anthology *Nurse Case Management in the 21st Century*, describes future nursing roles to include an increased emphasis on:

• Advocacy
• Learning

- Collaboration
- Coaching
- Resource management for groups and other care providers

Some of the nursing competencies needed for these roles include:

- Critical thinking
- Flexibility
- Relational skills for collaborative team practice
- Resource utilizing skills
- Information management skills
- Deep sensitivity for cultural diversity
- Community health and systems perspective

The March/April 1998 issue of *The American Nurse* points to some ways in which the statistics, trends, and predictions contained in this section are likely to translate into employment opportunities for nurses:

- A boom in home healthcare services for physically and/or mentally ill patients, increasing the need for general practice, high tech, and psychiatric home care nurses
- A need for critical care and emergency services, because critically ill patients will continue to be found all along the Continuum of Care. While nurses will continue to be used in great numbers in acute care hospitals, there will be a reduction from 68 percent to about 50 percent of all available practitioners to staff these settings, according to Tina Porter-O'Grady, who wrote the chapter, "Nurses as Advanced Practitioners and Primary Care Providers" in the anthology, *Nurse Case Management in the 21st Century*
- New employment opportunities related to an aging population, such as adult day care and assisted living centers
- Primary care and mental health services for school age children, including special needs children with tracheotomies, g-tubes, etcetera
- A higher volume of patients in ambulatory care centers needing sophisticated technical procedures
- Managed care companies as well as any healthcare organization focused on

economical, expedient, and safe access to and delivery of healthcare services. These compaies will use nurses to assess populations, determine health needs, plan programs of integrated health care, provide case management and utilization review, and provide telephone triage.

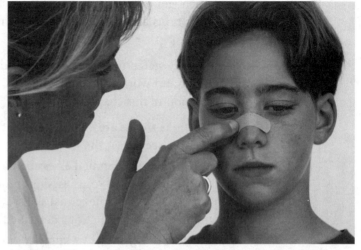

According to The American Nurse, *school-based care is a potential growth area in the years to come.*

- Increased opportunities for advanced practice registered nurses (APRN's), especially in the areas of gerontology and community-based psychiatry.

Where are the jobs most likely to be? According to the March/April 1998 issue of *The American Nurse*, some of the potential growth areas include:

- Home health
- Primary care
- Long-term care and other settings that serve older adults
- Critical and emergency care
- School-based care
- Outpatient care in hospitals
- Holistic nursing and alternative therapies
- Clinician, interventional coordinator and advanced roles in surgical settings
- Community settings, particularly in HMO-sponsored health promotion/disease prevention programs
- Ambulatory care

For additional discussion of how to interpret these statistics and apply them to potential employment options and opportunities, see chapter 7, "Product Development," and the appendix.

A prediction generally stated by futurists and trend watchers is that a change affecting the way you live and work will occur every six months! Therefore, to best make use of the information in this chapter:

- Explore how these trends are emerging and affecting actual employment situations you may be seeking at the time you intend to make a career change.
- Perform a self-initiated, biannual assessment of how (or whether) what you have to offer in the form of your nursing "product," expressed in the current state of your clinical and professional skills, is in alignment with the emergence of the trends and predictions described here.
- Use the appendix to expand your knowledge of healthcare trends and predictions that may be more specific to your chosen career path.

Employment Trends and Predictions

In 1994, the United States Department of Labor published the following statistics and predictions:

- An increased need for employment in service industries as opposed to manufacturing industries, with one out of three jobs in health, social services, and business. Health services alone are anticipated to experience an 89 percent growth rate.
- An additional 765,000 RNs (B.S.N.'s) will be required to meet the healthcare needs anticipated by the year 2005.
- Significant growth is anticipated between 1992 and 2005 in the following employment areas: computer and data processing, outpatient facilities and health services, personnel supply services (particularly home health attendants), health practitioners, child care services, legal services, nursing services, personal care services (including holistic modalities like massage), research services, management services, consulting services, residential care services, and business services (including credit reporting)

Each category of predicted employment growth above, contains a potential nursing role! Take a look:

Department of Labor Job Growth Predictions	Potential Nursing Role
Computer and data processing	Nurse informatics specialist
Outpatient facilities and health services	Occupational health nurse Ambulatory care nurse
Personnel supply services particularly home health attendants	Fee-for-service agency nurse assigned per diem to hospitals
Health practitioners	Adult nurse practitioner
Child care services	Pediatric nurse who establishes an after-school program for children with disabilities
Legal services	Legal nurse consultant
Nursing services	Direct care nurse
Personal care services, including holistic modalities like massage	Home care nurse with sub-specialty in pain management utilizing therapeutic touch, and imagery
Research, management, and consulting services	Nurse manager in an organizational reengineering consulting firm
Residential care services	Nurse in an assisted living center
Business services, including credit reporting	Nurse entrepreneur who opens a home care agency

Additional healthcare employment trends and predictions include:

- The age of the nation's RNs is increasing, with the average age in 1996 being 44, predicting a potential loss of seasoned nurses as they retire. By the year 2000, two thirds of all working RNs will be over age 40. In 1996, half of the California RN workforce was over the age of 45. That same year, the average age of the working RN in New York was 47. A possible balancing factor for this potential problem may be the aging of the Baby Boom generation, which is predicted to reinvent the retirement rules, opting for later retirement, with some deciding not to retire at all.

- There has been a decrease in nursing school enrollment since the early 1990s. Some experts believe that many potential nurses got scared away by what they erroneously believed to be a dismal forecast for the nursing job market as the Healthcare Revolution began and hospitals began downsizing. Other factors affecting decreased enrollment include a broader array of career options available to the young women and men usually attracted to nursing.

To summarize, the consensus of opinion from a wide variety of experts is:

- Healthcare is a growth industry
- The need for skilled services will *increase* even though the venue of care changes
- The present nationwide shortage of skilled workers, including RN's, is expected to continue and most likely increase.

In order to make best use of these trends and predictions, another piece of data needs to be added to the mix and perhaps is best captured by the following *New York Times* (August 6, 1998) headline: "General Motors Plans to Build New, Efficient Assembly Plants: Would Need Fewer Workers, a Worry for Unions."

And, so it *seems* in healthcare, too: Fewer hospital nurses for sicker patients who stay for shorter periods of time, requiring a faster, more efficient way to diagnose, treat, and discharge them. Nurses, of course, can't be compared to auto workers any more than patients can be compared to automobiles—yet some workplace issues affect all industries, including healthcare. (The sensitive and hotly debated issues related to the safe and ethical care of patients in a managed-care environment are worthy of the kind of considered attention outside of the scope of this discussion. See the appendix for explorations of this important issue). The big difference, however, is that while both nurses and auto workers are being dislocated from traditional and familiar workplaces, the nurse has the advantage of continuing to do a version of what she has always done in another setting, if she is flexible and informed enough to *follow the patient, whose care is sure to continue* after discharge from the hospital. Just because a patient with head trauma, for example, spends five days in an acute care hospital (as compared to, perhaps, 10 days a few years ago) doesn't mean all of his healthcare needs were met during that time. It just means that he no longer meets the criteria for acute care established by hospitals in response to managed care companies. This patient will receive a continuation of care elsewhere. When you understand how this Continuum of Care works, you have a road map you can use to find your place in the many employment sectors contained within it.

Employment Opportunities Along the Continuum of Care

The Continuum of Care is a framework for the delivery of healthcare services in a primary-care environment, with a focus on health as well as illness and injury. The phrase refers to the process by which the patient will receive healthcare services along a pathway that spans the gamut between wellness and prevention of illness on one end, to rehabilitation or long term care on the other end, taking into consideration levels of patient acuity occurring at any point along the way. The Continuum of Care represents a paradigm shift, a change in the mental map that is used to define or describe something in a particular way. In this case, it's a shift from the problem-oriented medical model of diagnosis and cure to the perspective of holism and prevention, with an emphasis on self-care.

Prior to the Healthcare Revolution, the hospital was the focal point of patient care, as well as employment for nurses. According to the Future Needs Project of the American Nurses Association, the hospital remains the largest employment setting for nurses, although its ranks are decreasing, from 67 percent in 1992 to 60 percent in 1996, with dramatic increases occurring in non-hospital employment settings. As a result of our restructured healthcare system, we are shifting away from this costly acute care option to a broader array of venues. *Nursing,* a Montefiore Medical Center Newsletter, captured the meaning and impact of the Continuum of Care by stating, "The Healthcare System is no longer a hospital, but rather a vertically integrated system made up of entities across a broad Continuum of Care. The Continuum of Care today is not from the day of admission to the day of discharge. *It is from the time of birth to the time of death.*" Remember, nobody has downsized accidents, illnesses, births, or deaths—only jobs! And, the jobs that are most affected are those in one segment of the Continuum of Care, namely, the Acute Care Hospital . . . another indisputable fact to circulate within the marketplace research department of You, Inc.

Along the Continuum of Care are the healthcare options for patients, as well as the employment opportunities for the nurse of today and tomorrow. To find the best employment opportunities even as the healthcare marketplace shuffles and reshuffles itself, watch the societal, cultural, and employment trends and predictions affecting healthcare and monitor the activities of the healthcare facilities along this Continuum of Care. Conduct research on what facilities and services are affected and how. As services develop, and the patient proceeds along this continuum, so do your employment options. For purposes of this discussion, the Continuum of Care will be divided into (1) acute care hospitals, (2) postacute care facilities and services, (3) additional community-based settings, and (4) supporting and affiliating services and facilities.

Acute-Care Hospitals

Acute care hospitals are what most people think of when they consider the need for inpatient healthcare. This is the type of hospital where most people think they will go when sick or injured, and where they may still believe they will stay until they are well. Though it's among the most familiar of the facilities along the Continuum of Care, it's also the most changed.

What has changed most in this setting is the rapid turnover of sicker patients, along with a technological explosion, not only in the clinical areas, but throughout the entire workplace, cutting across every job function. Most experts agree that while the need for acute care services will continue, only the sickest of the sick, requiring the most sophisticated technological support and intervention, will be cared for here.

This means that the kind of work for nurses in this setting will revolve around short-term relationships with very sick patients in an extremely high-tech environment.

Another significant change affecting nurses as acute care hospitals redesign their patient care delivery systems is the role of RNs, whose work assignments typically reflect a higher nurse-patient ratio. They are now asked to supervise unlicensed assistive personnel in the performance of skills and tasks once reserved only for the professional nurse, or perhaps the licensed practical nurse. The effect of this change on safe and effective patient care delivery is and should be of great concern to nurses who are mandated to be patient advocates as part of their legal license to practice nursing. In considering employment in acute-care hospitals, you need to carefully evaluate these issues, determining if this setting, as it changes, is most aligned with your vision, values, and mission. In addition, you should determine for yourself, directly or through informational interviewing, if the acute care hospital for which you are considering employment has restructured in ways that do not support safe and effective nursing care. Not all acute care hospitals have cut nursing care services so drastically that patient care is in jeopardy. In fact, the basic premise for organizational restructuring is to increase efficiency, and this includes freeing the professional nurse from non-nursing tasks. Some hospitals have done or are attempting to do this quite well. This is an unfinished issue to be closely monitored by each individual nurse, just as it is monitored by the American Nurses Association and each state nurses' association, as well. See Appendix A for additional information and guidance regarding this issue.

Post-Acute Care Facilities and Services

Post-acute care services are among the fastest growing sectors along this pathway and include the following kinds of facilities:

- Transitional care hospitals
- Subacute care facilities
- Long-term care facilities (previously called nursing homes)
- Assisted living facilities
- Home healthcare services
- Adult daycare services

Transitional Hospitals

These facilities, which are new on the Care Continuum with only about 120 in the United States today, provide longer-term care for critically ill patients who are in stable condition. The patients in these facilities require intensive, skilled care from a wide variety of healthcare disciplines, with the average, minimum stay around 25 days. Following his horseback riding accident, actor Christopher Reeve was cared for in a transitional hospital after he was somewhat stabilized in an acute care hospital.

Because the transitional hospital doesn't have to fund services typically found in acute-care hospitals, such as ambulatory clinics and emergency departments, they can provide a broad range of acute care interventions, including ICU-type services at about one-third to one-half the cost of acute care hospitals. This, of course, makes them quite attractive to managed-care companies. Rather than duplicate such services as lab and X-ray, they purchase them when needed from affiliated agencies, thereby avoiding the costly purchase and maintenance of these services.

Sub-Acute Care Facilities

The patient requiring care in sub-acute facilities falls somewhere between needing less intensive care than an acute-care hospital would provide but more than what the long-term facility can offer. This, along with rehabilitation, makes for a unique combination of services. The care provided is short-term (average length of stay is five to fourteen days), with a focused plan geared to helping the patient achieve a specific goal, for example, walk independently with a cane following hip replacement surgery. The patient is then referred to the next place along the Care Continuum, as indicated. These patients are stable, but can still be quite ill, often requiring high-tech monitoring. As in the transitional hospital, they receive skilled interventions from a multidisciplinary team.

Long-Term Care Facilities

The change in name from *nursing homes* to *long-term care facilities* reflects the influence of changing economics and reimbursement mechanisms. These facilities restructured their services in response to the need to provide a higher level of skilled intervention for their patients when they become ill, rather than transferring them to a more costly facility like acute care hospitals. In addition to becoming the extension of the patient's family and community that it has always been, the long-term care facility now has an increasing number of specialty units, all designed to treat the patient while ill, including care for patients with dementia.

Hospice Services

The majority of hospice services are part of and administered by home care programs, or by inpatient facilities along the Continuum of Care, such as the acute-care hospital, in collaboration with visiting nurses. Hospice care provides a variety of services and support to terminally ill patients, generally with a prognosis of six months or less to live, including skilled nursing care, home health aides and attendants, and specialized medical equipment as indicated. The combined focus on physical care and emotional support is frequently described by hospice nurses as both challenging and rewarding.

Assisted Living Facilities

This new and mostly privately funded addition to the Continuum of Care provides several levels of healthcare and personal care services for the well-elderly who want to live independently, as well as special facilities for the frail elderly. Other groups, such as the physically or emotionally disabled, are starting to take advantage of this new option. Assisted living facilities offer apartment-style living along with such personal support services as dining room meals, often served in attractive restaurant-like atmospheres, household cleaning and repair, and recreational activities. The residents enjoy the benefits of security, companionship, and access to ongoing healthcare, or, when necessary, immediate emergency care. Healthcare, ambulatory as well as inpatient, is provided through a network of affiliating agencies, often representing all the options along the Care Continuum. Even patients with dementia and Alzheimer's disease can be accommodated in the specialized units of some assisted living facilities.

Home Healthcare Services

Technological advances as well as economic constraints have fostered a growth boom in home healthcare services. This is believed to be the fastest growing segment of the healthcare marketplace, with high-tech and psychiatric home care growing the fastest.

Today's home care patient tends to be more severely and chronically ill than ever before. Home care agencies fall into three general categories: licensed, certified, and long-term. The licensed agencies provide private-duty nursing as well as assistive and personal care support, often from home health attendants. The certified agencies care for sicker patients, often those discharged "quicker and sicker" from the acute care hospital, and offer a broad range of services such as rehabilitation, assistance in daily living activities from home health aides, and social service support. Long-term home care agencies provide supportive care to those patients who are chronically ill and qualify for a long-term inpatient care facility but who chose to remain at home.

Adult Day Care Services

These facilities provide skilled nursing, assisted personal care, and long-term care to patients that may or may not be receiving simultaneous home care services. Patients come to day care for socialization or for such skilled nursing services as insulin monitoring and tracheostomy care. These facilities provide the patients with an enhanced quality of life, and the caregiver-relative with an excellent option for rest and relief, or even just the freedom to do errands or go to work.

Additonal Community-Based Settings

In addition to the post-acute care employment options discussed above, and attempting to keep pace with the reduction of acute-care beds, are the redesigned and ever-increasing variety of familiar healthcare services and facilities outside the traditional acute care hospital walls. These services include:

- Ambulatory healthcare centers, including physician or nurse-based practices, free-standing or hospital-based clinics, and health maintenance organizations for all healthcare specialties, including mental health and substance abuse
- Ambulatory surgicenters
- Occupational and corporate healthcare services and wellness programs found in most traditional workplaces as well as more exotic locations like movie sets, circuses, sporting events, concerts, resorts, camps, spas, health clubs, and weight loss centers
- Family planning centers

- Birthing centers
- Pain management centers
- Wound care centers
- Hemodialysis centers
- Outreach centers of churches, synagogues, and other religious institutions
- Forensic and prison healthcare services and facilities
- School health offices and centers
- Shelters, housing assistance, and mobile crisis programs for the homeless and mentally ill

Supporting and/or Affiliating Services and Territories

Completing most of the picture of the healthcare employment territories that relate directly or indirectly to the Continuum of Care are the following types of facilities, services, institutions, and organizations. These form a web of support that serves and/or associates with the Continuum of Care, including the education of healthcare personnel, and which represents the for-profit and nonprofit sectors. Interesting employment options exist for nurses in all of these areas.

- Pharmaceutical and medical supply companies. These companies hire nurses to market their products to a variety of healthcare settings. Responsibilities might include teaching skills related to the product (such as the use of specialized dressings for wound care) and providing information to primary care providers.
- Healthcare consulting organizations. These include a vast array of services and programs including computer consulting, organizational redesign firms, and human resource consulting.
- Personnel supply organizations, of professional and ancillary, per diem and private duty staff for inpatient and community-based settings
- Schools of nursing education for basic, undergraduate, and graduate education, as well as continuing education

Potential Nursing Roles Along the Continuum of Care

Now that you are armed with a map of healthcare's new, revised, and traditional territories, the next task for the market research department of You, Inc., is to consider the potential nursing roles associated with them. A partial list, including a brief overview of these roles, is provided below. Recommendations for a more comprehensive description of these and many other nursing roles can be found in Appendix A.

The three basic roles of clinician, manager, and educator can be found just about anywhere along the Continuum of Care, with more and more interesting combinations, options, and opportunities emerging every day. Each of these three basic nursing roles (See chapter 7, "Product Development," for a more extensive discussion of them) can include all levels of competence, from novice to expert, with nursing practice options as a generalist (in medical-surgical nursing, for example) as well as a specialist (in gerontology or psychiatry, for example). In the examples on the next page, remember that the roles of clinician, manager, and educator overlap tremendously and are only separated here for clarity.

Another helpful way to determine where to take your nursing service or "product" is to know what the work responsibilities and expectations are in the nursing venue or role you are considering. This will help you to find the best match between you and it. Extremely effective methods of obtaining this data include informational interviewing, networking, and, of course, during employment interviews.

As you review some of the typical work expectations and responsibilities outlined below, keep in mind the overlapping of responsibilities that is bound to occur among the different settings.

Basic Nursing Role	Example of Nursing Practice Option	Potential Place of Employment among the Continuum of Care
Manager or educator	Nurse informatics specialist	All settings
Educator	Nursing school faculty	Colleges, schools, continuing education sites
Manager	Nurse case manager Risk manager Utilization reviewer	Inpatient settings Community settings Insurance companies
Clinician	Patient advocate	Inpatient settings
Clinician	Telephone triage nurse	Insurance companies Managed care companies Hospital ERs
Clinician	Parish nurse	Churches, religious centers
Clinician, manager, or educator	Nurse consultant	All settings Private practice
Clinician, manager, or educator	Nurse attorney Legal nurse consultant Paralegal nurse	Private practice Attorney's offices Risk management departments in all settings
Clinician, manager, or educator	Nurse entrepreneur	Private practice in psychotherapy Owner of home care agency
Clinician	Advanced practice nurse Nurse practitioner direct care nurse specialist	Nurse-run clinic Nurse-physician group practice All settings as primary care provider for NP

Facility	Responsibilites And Expectations
Acute care hospitals	Fast-paced action
	Extremely fluid environment
	Rapid patient turnover
	Short-term nurse-patient relationship
	High nurse-patient ratio
	High tech environment
Post-acute care inpatient settings	Longer-term patient relationships
	Combined ICU-type skills with routine medical-surgical intervention
	Strong emphasis on teaching and patient self-care
Ambulatory care settings	High volume of patients in short periods of time
	Triage and prioritizing skills essential
	Strong emphasis on patient teaching
Home care settings	Creative in solving unexpected problems
	Independent and self-reliant
	Flexible scheduling
	Regular involvement with patient's family, others
	Excellent organizational skills
	Strong emphasis on teaching, support, self-care

New Nursing Practice Options and Opportunities

Some of the newer or expanded nursing practice options include but are not limited to the following:

- Nurse informatics specialist
- Nurse case manager
- Nurse executive
- Advanced nurse practitioner (direct care nurse specialist or nurse practitioner)

- Ethics consultant
- Nurse career strategist
- Nurse entrepreneur

See the appendix for information on these and other nursing practice opportunities.

Summary

Given the array of options and opportunities described in this section, it's hard to imagine not being able to find employment in the traditional and emerging territories in the Healthcare Frontier. This is not to say it is always easy, given the volatility of the changing marketplace. A key to success is playing the workplace game by the new rules discussed throughout this book and by other career strategists, and briefly reviewed here as you ponder your career path along the healthcare industry's Continuum of Care:

- Work towards and preserve your first-class ticket to ride, your front-row seat in the theater of healthcare employment. This includes a B.S.N. degree, ANCC or other professional board certification at the generalist or specialist levels, current and relevant continuing education, and broad cross-training.
- Stay loose and flexible. Be prepared to move to what's new and what's next, managing the stress of change that may accompany it, or perhaps learning to revel in the adventure of it, as you thrive rather than just manage to survive.
- Take your role as the chief executive and chief managing officer of You, Inc. seriously. Manage your career as if it was your own business by organizing the activities in all the departments of You, Inc. in ways that stay in alignment with the best employment options possible.
- Revise, revise, and revise again. Keep the root of the word *revise* in mind: It means to look over something, or to correct or improve, to make a new version of; it means to review, take another look, update. Keep working on your vision, values and mission. They are sure to change as you change, certain to need reshaping as you are reshaped by the work experiences you have along your career path.

Chapter 9

Developing a Marketing Plan

Successful business owners know that a well-developed marketing plan is essential in helping them identify which customers are most likely to be attracted to their venture. Your marketing plan can put a foundation under your vision and translate your hopes and dreams into reality by establishing goals and tasks necessary to move you along your chosen

> "Listening to your heart is not simple. Finding out who you are is not simple. It takes a a lot of hard work and courage to get to know who you are and what you want."
> —Sue Bender

career path. It reflects the special attributes of the work you do and helps you identify where it might be most needed. Your marketing plan can help you determine the match between your marketable skills and the marketplace needs. It takes the data and ideas generated from the Product Development, Marketplace Research, Advertising, Sales, and Networking Departments of You, Inc. and pulls them together into a coherent whole, a cohesive document, a place for you to focus your energy.

A prime reason for creating a marketing plan is for the clarity that results. It will either confirm the validity of the path you have chosen or lead you to rethink it, thereby saving you valuable time, energy, and resources. As stated in earlier chapters, you should expect to rethink or at least validate the continued marketability of your career path about every six months.

A good marketing plan is a roadmap, a time schedule, and a feedback mechanism all rolled into one. Add to this a measure of focused commitment, periodically mixed with the support and encouragement of the people in your network and mentoring system, and you have a solid recipe for success and career resilience.

To develop your marketing plan, follow the steps below, which are borrowed from the business world and translated into concepts relevant to your nursing career path. Fill in the blanks as they relate to your experience, and/or to the career goals you are considering. Feel free to add other sections to personalize this plan for your situation.

Step 1: Describe Your Mission, Your Values, and Your Vision

This self-management step is essential if you want to find the best employment match for your skills and experience. It will also minimize the burnout associated with feeling trapped in a job with which you are not aligned. You will need to recall the following three qualities you worked on in chapter 7, "Product Development."

Your mission statement _____

_____

_____

Your professional and personal values _____

_____

_____

Your vision statement _____

_____

_____

Step 2: Select Your Business

The business you are in is expressed by the overall nursing role you perform. As discussed in chapter 7, "Product Development," your nursing role is a blending of basic work skills and core nursing competencies. Follow the steps below to identify what your preferred nursing role is. This is the "business" you are currently in.

Basic Work Skills

1. Reflect on your present job, or one you may be considering.

2. List all the work skills and activities that this job requires.

_____

_____

3. Which skills and activities do you:

like to do? _____

dislike doing?_____

want to do more of?_____

4. Refer to the general categories of basic work skills below. Which do you prefer to spend the most time doing? Rank them in your order of preference with 1 signifying "most preferred" and 3 signifying "least preferred":

_____ People skills

_____ Data and information skills

_____ Concept and idea skills

Core Nursing Competencies

1. Refer to the discussion of core nursing competencies in the product development chapter and the list below.

2. Which do you prefer to spend the most time doing?

3. Rank them in your order of preference with 1 = most preferred and 5 = least preferred:

_____ Clinical competencies

_____ Managerial competencies

_____ Educational competencies

_____ Interpersonal competencies

_____ Technical competencies

Your Preferred Nursing Role

The business you are currently in is: _____

An example of this role is: _____

Where a nurse in this example might work is (see chapter 8, "Marketplace Research"):

_____

Step 3: Assess Your Level of Nursing Practice Proficiency

Using Benner's model as described in the chapter 7, "Product Development," identify the level of nursing practice proficiency you have now, or the level that's expected in the role you are considering.

- ❒ Level I = Novice
- ❒ Level II = Advanced Beginner
- ❒ Level III = Competent
- ❒ Level IV = Proficient
- ❒ Level V = Expert

Step 4: Select a Healthcare Territory

Identify an employment option or territory you would like to target by analyzing and reviewing the traditional and emerging territories along the Continuum of Care, as described in the chapter 8, "Marketplace Research," as well in other sources.

Consider the geographical location most attractive to you as well as those locations that most likely contain your target market. Determine what employment and/or cultural trends and predictions might affect your choice. For example, the downsizing of acute care hospitals is negatively influencing the hiring of new B.S.N. graduates in many, but not all, areas of the country.

Identify who your customer is, meaning the employer who is most likely to want what you have to offer. For example, the customer of the new B.S.N. graduate might be a large medical center with a strong staff development department and an internship program. Or, it might be a community hospital in which an associate degree graduate performed clinical rotations.

Fill in the following answers from the work you did in chapter 7, "Product Development."

Your target market is: _____

Your customer is: _____

Related societal and cultural trends are: _____

_____

Related employment trends are: _____

_____

Qualifications for this target market are: _____

_____

Are you currently qualified?

❏ Yes

❏ No (rethink what you need to do)

❏ Perhaps, if . . . (specify what you need to do and see step 6 below)

Step 5: Research the Competition and Know How to Stand Out

No business owner who intends to succeed would ever think of investing time, money, or other resources in a service or product without an awareness of who else was doing it and how they match up against them. Neither should you. The way to compete most effectively is to know how to stand out so you don't fade out!

Answer the following questions:

How is your service (what you have to offer) as good as or better than the service of others who have the same or a similar nursing "business?"

_____

_____

_____

_____

If you, along with 50 other nurses, applied for the job you want, what would make you at least as qualified, or even more qualified?

_____

_____

_____

_____

What value do you add to the mission of the organization where you are seeking employment (or in which you are currently working) as compared to the others also seeking it or working within it?

_____

_____

_____

_____

In what ways would you improve the quality of the service the organization provides, beyond the minimum requirement of showing up for work and performing the tasks required in your job description?

_____

_____

_____

_____

Taking Stock

Review the lists below. On a scale of 1 to 5 (see below), how would you rate your ability to compete effectively?

1 = unable to compete effectively

2 = need work to compete effectively

3 = able to compete under some circumstances

4 = able to compete fairly well, in most circumstances

5 = able to compete effectively

Professional Experience

_____ Targeted, progressive, cumulative work as a generalist and a specialist

_____ Has examples of "value-added" work experiences

_____ Aware of, able to support, and can contribute to patient-focused care in a consumer-oriented business environment

_____ Diverse, transferable skills

_____ Cross-training

_____ Continuing education

_____ Computer literate and Internet savvy

_____ Bachelor of Science in Nursing

_____ Advanced educational preparation commensurate with career goals

_____ ANCC board-certification as a generalist or specialist (or other professional certification)

_____ Professional membership

_____ Additional: _____

Personal Characterics

_____ Flexible, adaptive, assertive, confident, empowered

_____ Self-directed and team savvy

_____ Innovative problem solver

_____ Does not accept status quo

_____ Willing to take risks

_____ Learns from mistakes

_____ Conflict resolver

_____ Critical thinker

_____ Master networker

_____ Additional: _____

Note: This is by no means a complete list. It provides some examples that contribute to effective professional practice and employment in a competitive healthcare marketplace. Feel free to add to this list, personalizing it to your situation.

Step 6: Identify Needs and Resources

The business meaning of the term _resources_ has been expanded from its usual focus on financial resources. For the purposes of your marketing plan as a nurse, it includes all of the personal and interpersonal resources that are necessary to achieve your goal, including the potential obstacles and competing priorities that might exist. Consider the needs and resources identified below as they relate to the "business" you selected and the market you targeted. Then fill in the blanks.

Current, transferable skills (include non-nursing work)

_____

_____

Strengths and vulnerabilities, professional, personal (selling points or areas needing work)

_____

_____

Priorities (competing personal and professional situations)

_____

_____

Potential obstacles (personal and professional)

_____

_____

Inner barriers (limiting beliefs such as "I'm too old, too young, too busy"_____

_____

Outer obstacles (such as lack of experience or credentials)

_____

_____

Training and education needs

_____

_____

Insurance, licensure, certification needs and issues

_____

_____

Networking needs (see chapter 10, "Networking")

_____

_____

Professional network: list key names

_____

_____

Personal network: list key names

_____

_____

Networking activities and events to target for attending

_____

_____

Advertising needs: status of your résumé

    ❐ Nonexistent

    ❐ Needs revision. Comments: _____

    ❐ Updated and ready

Professional portfolio

    ❐ Nonexistent

    ❐ Needs revision. Comments: _____

    ❐ Updated and ready

Selling strategies: status of your interviewing skills

    ❐ Satisfactory

    ❐ Needs work. Comments: _____

Financial needs and issues, including sources of revenue if applicable

_____

_____

Stress management and self care needs

_____

_____

Additional issues and considerations

_____

_____

After considering all of the needs and resources you have just reviewed, What do you already have in place? What needs to be added? Where will you get what you need?

Step 7: Determine Your Risk Potential and Risk Tolerance

Risk tolerance is a financial term that refers to the difference between what you have contributed to your venture—your personal investment—as compared with what others have contributed or invested.

The more you invest in yourself, financially and in all other ways, the more freedom and control you have over your own business and its direction, in this case, your nursing practice. "Control" is key here, and has direct implications for You, Inc., especially in these times of constant change and permanent transition. The more you are in charge of your own resources, such as networks outside of your workplace, tuition reimbursement, and even (when possible) health insurance, the freer you are to make decisions related to the direction of your "business."

Taking advantage of employment benefits and using the resources of your employer is wonderful and useful _to the degree that it does not deter you from your mission_, or transfer the control of You, Inc. out of your hands, steering you in an unwanted direction. Sometimes this happens out of necessity, because of limited resources or competing priorities, like having small children, for example. While there are certainly times when the priority needs to be employment benefits over career direction and control, there are also times when both can occur. However, the more you believe in your ability to provide for this on your own, the more your actions will prove you true. What's important here is your awareness of what you are doing and why, so that you do not get lulled into complacency and stuck in a job you hate because the benefits are too good to give up.

Determine your risk potential by estimating the percentage of investment you are making, as compared with the investment of others (most especially your employer). The higher the percentage of your own investment, the lower the risk of losing control of your professional direction.

Percentage of resources contributed by you (rough estimate) _____

Percentage of resources contributed by employer (rough estimate) _____

Profit and Loss Analysis

This term is used by business owners to denote a method of assessing overall financial risk. Here it is translated to mean the overall risk to be found in your selected career step, after weighing all the pros and cons.

Pros of following this career path (reasons to pursue): _____

_____

Cons of following this career path (reasons not to pursue): _____

_____

How I will profit from this career step is: _____

_____

What I might lose is: _____

_____

To determine how tolerable the risk is, consider the following risk factors. Using the Risk-Safety Scale below, rank them on the following scale.

Risk-Safety Scale

1 = very safe	5 = more risky than safe
2 = mostly safe	6 = somewhat risky
3 = somewhat safe	7 = mostly risky
4 = more safe than risky	8 = very risky

Score   Risk factors

_____   Financial costs, personal and professional

_____   Effect of career goal on competing priorities

_____   Capacity to manage the stress of change

_____   Relative stability of the market territory you are targeting

_____   Additional personal or professional considerations

After analyzing the data from the previous two scores, and using the same risk-safety scale, your overall risk tolerance for this career step is: _____

Is this career path feasible?

❏ Yes

❏ No (rethink what you need to do)

❏ Perhaps, if _____

Step 8: Identify Your Goal and Create a Plan

This is where you activate your marketing plan by identifying your goal and then creating a plan to make it happen.

Goal Setting

Identify a goal and write it below in specific and concrete terms. The more specific you are, the easier it will be to develop a plan to make it happen. Use action verbs and events that can be measured or seen. For example, *finding a job as a nurse* is not as specific or measurable as *finding work as a med-surg nurse in a tertiary care medical center of at least 800 beds within 3 months.*

Tasks and Target Dates

Next, identify the tasks you need to do for the goal to be achieved. For the example above, this may include updating your résumé, among other things. Again, make the task as specific as possible, breaking it into its smallest components. The process of getting the résumé written may have many steps within it; for example, finding your old résumé, talking to friends about their résumés, and making an appointment with a résumé writer. Each task should have a target date of completion to keep you on track. Try using the sheet on the next page to organize this information.

Evaluation and Revisions

It is often necessary to revise your goals. This may not be evident until action is taken and you begin to evaluate the results. Keeping track of your progress in this way will lead you to revisions as necessary. As you move along, it may become clear that the entire goal of mounting a job search is totally mistimed and needs to be delayed for awhile. Or you may discover that the target dates were too ambitious and while the goal is still feasible, you need to adjust the task list and target dates more realistically.

GOAL #1: _____

_____

_____

Tasks (what actions are needed?)	Target Dates (by when?)	Outcomes (evaluate the results and identify what's next)	Revisions (develop new goals and/or tasks, as needed

Search Strategies

Now that you have a marketing plan specifying what you have to offer, it's time to find those who might be interested in it. The more scheduled time you are willing to devote to your work search, the more it will pay off for you. In the current, competitive job market, depending on what kind of work you are looking for, you might discover that finding a new job is practically a full time job in and of itself. There is more to do than just send out a résumé and wait for a response, as previous chapters in this book have described. Some tips to keep you on track include:

- Set aside time each day to track your progress.
- Create a space in your home to keep the supplies and information you need to accomplish this task. Consider including some motivational or inspirational material in the form of quotes, pictures, or symbols to encourage you.
- Keep track of your progress, in writing.
- Start a folder or develop a filing system for each employer contact you have made and note the time of the next contact, the result of the contact, your impressions of the conversation, and what the next step is.
- Think twice before sending out résumés and query letters to potential employers who may not be looking for what you have to offer. This kind of "shotgun" approach can disperse your energy, especially if time is short. Each letter you send requires follow-up contact of some sort, making this a very time-intensive way to search for a job. On the other hand, the payoff could be big if you are seeking a job that is not often advertised or is otherwise hard to find.

There are many work search methods from which to choose. These include:

Resources Within Your Present Organization

During organizational restructuring, there is often a loss of nurses or nursing roles during restructuring, but that loss is accompanied by the creation of new, redesigned ways in which nurses will work, resulting in new employment opportunities. Have your résumé ready. Be prepared to be interviewed as if you were being hired from outside the organization. Network for the information you'll need to gain a competitive edge.

The Internet

Online resources for employment information and job listings can be useful as well as time consuming, depending on the status of your computer skills and the speed of your modem and Internet connection. Use this source to supplement what you already know. Keep track of its growing importance as technology improves and its use permeates the mainstream employment and networking cultures. Cynthia Saver in *Searching the Internet for Jobs and Career Advice* describes four types of career information available on the Internet:

- Career advice
- Labor market websites for economic, labor, and industry trends
- Online job listings, including electronic résumé submission
- Company information

Additional employment resources include:

- All print media such as newspapers and nursing journals
- Networking and employment publications such as *Nursing Spectrum*
- Networking events, including seminars, conventions, and job fairs

Networking is one of the best work search methods and is explored in the following chapter.

Chapter 10

Networking

Networks are loose, fluid, dynamic webs of personal and professional alliances forged for the purpose of sharing knowledge, exchanging information, and providing support. Networks are everywhere people are. They can spontaneously emerge or you can create them on purpose. You can take them with you, leave

> "The good life is a process, not a state of being. It is a direction, not a destination."
> —Carl Rogers

them behind, form new ones, merge old and new networks, or create formal and informal networks. Professional or personal networks can extend your reach, encourage your vision, strengthen your resolve, and bolster your strength.

The currency of exchange in this Age of Information is communication and knowledge. Network relationships provide the way to exchange this currency, as well as make it grow. Because nurses are knowledge workers, and knowledge constantly increases, networks become essential links to and repositories of vast amounts of knowledge and information that you alone could never completely acquire or keep current. Allowing your networks to hold some of this information until you need it frees your mind, and is a smart strategy for dealing with the stress of information overload. In this way, networks can become knowledge and information storehouses, awaiting a time when you need what's in it.

This description of *networks* extends their meaning and purpose far beyond what comes to the mind of most people who might only associate them with job searching. Just like a computer is not simply a complex typewriter, so is networking more complex than just a job search mechanism.

A network represents the connections between and among people and systems; some with direct relationships to one another, and others like cousins are once or twice removed. You may not know the person who has the knowledge or information you need, but if your network is large enough, you can be "one or two degrees of separation" from obtaining it. In *Effective Networking*, Venda Raye-Johnson describes a study done by Milgram that demonstrates the reality of this. She asked a group of people in Massachusetts to use the contacts in their networks to reach a group of people unknown to them in Nebraska that he had randomly selected. The people in Massachusetts were able to reach the randomly selected group in Nebraska within two contacts. Here is an example of how this can work in nursing:

Joan is a medical surgical staff nurse with an associate degree, currently enrolled in a B.S.N. program. She has four years of oncology nursing experience and is considering becoming board-certified as an oncology nurse. She wonders about the pros and cons, who offers certification, how others nurses feel about it, and how it might have benefited them. She asks four people she knows about it: two nurse colleagues at work, the professor teaching her class at school, and the woman she just met, sitting next to her on the bus going home, who turns out to be a nurse. The schematic diagram on the next page demonstrates how networks function and what Joan was able to learn as a result.

As you can see from the diagram, not only did Joan get the information she needed, she was able to obtain her certification while she still met the eligibility requirements, a side benefit she hadn't anticipated. Notice that she had tiered links to information, with some sources "once removed" (two degrees of separation) and others "twice removed" (three degrees of separation). Joan may never meet the people who provided the beneficial information that she needed. Likewise, those people may also one day benefit from information Joan has.

The Benefits of Participating in Networks

Consider establishing or joining a professional or personal network if you need to:

- Track professional and employment trends
- Find role models and mentors
- Enhance your vision, your future goals, allowing it to develop as you grow ready to implement it

JOAN'S NETWORK

JOAN
Needs information about certification: Why, where, when, and how.

Person #5
"You can borrow my certification catalog.".

Person #6
"I got certified last year."

Person #1
"I saw a help-wanted ad for an oncology nurse and certification was a preferred qualification."

Person #2
"The oncology nurse certification is called OCN, I think. "

Person #3
"This is the last year nurses who don't have a B.S.N. can get certified."

Person #4
"I saw an article about it in last month's AJN."

Person #7
"ANCC provides certification at two levels: generalist and specialist."

Person #8
"My sister just got her OCN certification. Here's her phone number."

Person #9
"A friend at work just got certified."

Person #10
"When possible, I hire only certified nurses."

Person #11
"I teach review courses for certification exams."

Person #12
"I just took the certification review courses. I'll give you the sign-up information."

Person #13
"A big factor in landing this job was my certification"

Person #14
"I know how to get certified."

- Receive support, feedback, or encouragement
- Learn new skills or build transferable skills
- Search for a job by obtaining leads about work opportunities, asking for recommendations and conducting informational interviews
- Experience the satisfaction of passing along your own knowledge, skills, and information
- Feel good about supporting or mentoring others
- Relax through the diversion of play or humor

Places to Look For Networking Opportunities

Wherever there are people, you will find networks which are already established, or the candidates for them. A partial list of places follows. Can you think of others relevant in your life?

- Work relationships, present and former
- School relationships, present and former
- Professional associations
- Conventions, seminars, conferences
- Relationships with your personal physician, dentist, accountant, and/or lawyer
- Friends and neighbors
- Health and sports clubs, or any other kinds of social clubs

Networking Skills and Strategies

Be Assertive and Proactive

Take the initiative to establish conversations. If this is not your strength, use networking to learn and develop it, perhaps by seeking out a mentor, coach, or role model you can emulate. The networking experience itself will provide the practice; you just need to provide the motivation, commitment, and patience.

Present Yourself with Confidence

Create and rehearse a brief introduction of who you are, a summary of your professional experience and/or personal interests. Consider an achievement of yours that others would be interested in, especially if it is relevant to the networking topic. In addition, take care about the image you are communicating by dressing professionally or appropriately for the occasion.

Formalize the Networking Experience

While networks are often informal social links, your approach to the process itself should be formalized. The more effort you put into it and structure you create around it, the more you will get out of it. Ways to formalize networking include:

- Conducting research to determine which networks would best suit your needs.
- Setting a goal to introduce yourself and initiate a conversation with at least 5–10 people at every networking event you attend.
- Preparing a business card to exchange with others. It creates an impressive image, and is also a way to keep track of who you meet.
- Establishing a record-keeping system, such as a card file to use when needed.

Increase Your Visibility

Attend meetings, join organizations, volunteer, work on committees. Remember that networking is a mutual experience and exchange. Don't go to events just to see what may be in it for you. The more you put into the experience, the more you will get out of it. When possible, work on shaping it to meet your needs rather than complaining that it doesn't work for you. If this kind of proactive approach does not work, consider joining other network sources.

Practice Active Listening

Because networking is about mutuality, about giving and getting, be a good listener, not just a talker. Try listening twice as much as you speak, as this anonymous quote reminds us: "God gave us two ears and one mouth, so we should listen twice as much as we speak!"

Consider Everyone You Meet a Contact

See the world anew, as a vast pool of networking possibilities. Smile, strike up conversations, look for opportunities to exchange information and seek opportunities. As the CEO of You, Inc., take responsibility for the operational well-being of your company seriously by being ever-ready to promote yourself and support others.

Open Windows When Doors Close

Transform rejection into potential opportunity whenever possible. For example, the Nurse Recruiter who didn't give you the job you wanted closed the door. Try opening a window of opportunity by keeping in touch with her, maybe sending updated résumés periodically. Or consider striking up conversations with her at professional meetings you may be at together. In this way, she can become a link in your network, perhaps a connection to other work situations.

Trust the Process

Make networking an adventure by trusting that the links and connections in your network can eventually lead to opportunities that you may not yet be able to identify. Be optimistic by believing in a positive result, and keep the process going by attending meetings and nurturing relationships. However, trusting blindly in networking while you passively sit back waiting for something to happen is likely to get you nowhere. No amount of networking can compensate for a lack of attention to other aspects of You, Inc., such as product development, advertising, and sales.

Use the Grapevine

It is believed that 75 percent of the information circulated through gossip and rumor is actually founded in fact. However, since it is heavily peppered with the perceptions and interpretations of others, be sure to verify the information you get this way before acting on it. Consider some of it entertainment, perhaps like the game "telephone" you might have played as a child. Have fun with it, be careful with and about it, but at the same time, don't underestimate the power of it.

Network Electronically

Online networking is fast becoming one of the most important ways for knowledge workers like nurses to stay connected to professional sources of information. This can be done formally through Web sites of professional associations, or informally through chat rooms and list servers. While the format for networking online is quite different, the benefits and opportunities are the same. In addition, it eliminates the "not enough time" excuse, since it can be done at times that suit your schedule. See the appendix for some useful sites.

Chapter 11

Advertising

Writing Your Résumé

A résumé advertises the nature of your nursing "business," what your company of one, You, Inc., has to offer. It creates the opportunities needed for dialogues with potential employers/purchasers of your nursing services. A résumé is a sales tool that will not directly get you a job, but will open the door for you to make your pitch for it. It's the attention-getter you need to highlight your best features and accomplishments.

A résumé is a work in progress, an externalized representation of your professional nursing identity. As such, its style and content will grow and change over time, just as you do. There is a reassuring autobiographical quality to a well-written résumé that becomes almost like a mirror, reflecting where you have

> "You think you understand the situation, but what you don't understand is that the situation just changed."
>
> —An advertisement for Putnam Investments

been and what you have done while pointing the way to what you may do in the future. While employers may "own" your job and make decisions about its design and longevity, your résumé represents what *you* own; namely, *your* work, *your* achievements, and *your* experiences. It represents what belongs to you after leaving the particular job environment in which they occurred. As such, it can be a reminder of your career security in today's growth market.

Keep your résumé updated and ready for your next career step while doing the semiannual review of what you have to offer as the marketplace changes, as recommended in chapter 7, "Product Development." This will give you a degree of reassuring control and preparedness during the constant change and permanent transition typical of today's healthcare workplace.

A résumé is a *summary* of your experience and achievements, worded in short phrases. It is not a job description. It is not a complete description of everything you've done. In fact, a well-written résumé should create some questions—but not confusion—in the reader's mind, questions that could be asked of you in the interview. This gives you the opportunity to "sell," to convince the employer that you have the nursing skills, competencies, and experiences that they need. It allows you to emphasize the match between the employer and your abilities, and perhaps most importantly, to use the reactions of the interviewer to further shape your responses.

Periodically revising your résumé is a way to realign your professional identity, a way to remind yourself of where you've been and what your best experiences are (your bestselling features). The process of writing a résumé is likely to rescue from memory skills and achievements previously overlooked. Revisions also give you the opportunity to rephrase and therefore realign your skills with current marketplace needs, thereby making you more employable. Many such realignments can be expected along your nursing career path.

An excellent way to write or revise your résumé is to co-create it with someone who can provide feedback and objectivity and help you shape it into the best possible sales tool. Consider working with a friend or colleague who has good writing skills and who can to be objective about you. If you decide to use a professional résumé writer or career coach, be sure you are involved in co-creating it with them. Allowing someone else to produce the résumé in your absence denies you a level of involvement that serves to increase your confidence in You, Inc., in the professional identity which your résumé represents. If you choose to work on it alone, consider showing it to others for feedback.

Potential employers will be looking for a match between your credentials and experience on one hand and the requirements of the job needing to be filled on the other. Choose your words carefully and economically. Too many words, repetitions, or irrelevant data will work against you and may even eliminate you from the competition.

Résumé Appearance

Your résumé should be typed in a font typically used in business and professional documents such as Times Roman or Ariel. The size of the font should be 11 or 12 points. Avoid frilly, decorative fonts and use bolding, italics, and bullets sparingly. Pay close attention to any special instructions requested by potential employers who plan to scan your résumé into a computer. Since the computer cannot accurately scan anything decorative such as bullets or fancy fonts, ignoring these instructions may eliminate you from consideration. Generally, this is also true for résumés that are submitted online.

The résumé can be one to two pages in length, but never more than two. Set the margins of the paper so that the information can fill the page with enough white space (empty space surrounding the typed words) to make for easy reading. Absence of white space indicates an attempt to cram too much material into too small a space, and for this reason a two-page résumé, when necessary, is more advisable. It may indicate an attempt to write a more detailed description of your experience than is required in a résumé.

Use professional stationary with matching envelopes in white or off-white. It's acceptable to neatly handwrite the address on the envelope; in fact, a handwritten envelope may indicate a personal but still professional touch.

Keep in mind that there is no one way to write a résumé. After following the generally accepted guidelines presented here, it is a matter of personal preference. The type of résumé described here is called the reverse chronological résumé. An alternative is the skill-based résumé or some combination of both. Consult the appendix for more information, especially on how to write a skills-based résumé.

Résumé Preparation

1. Contact Information

Place your name, credentials, address, and phone number centered on the top of the page. A line that separates this identifying information from the remainder of the text provides a format style that makes reading easier and quicker. For example:

SALLY SMITH, B.S.N., R.N.

75 East Main Street, #7A

New York, NY 10010

(212) 555-9831

---

2. Profile or Summary of Qualifications

Use this in place of a job objective, which tends to limit and perhaps pigeonhole you. A job objective can be included in the cover letter that accompanies each résumé you send out. Guidelines for writing a cover letter are included at the end of this section.

You might wait until your résumé is completed to write the profile so that you have a better sense of what you want to include. A profile is a summary, not a complete repetition of your résumé. It should highlight your best "selling" features as well as the kind of characteristics that employers are looking for today.

Profile Examples

Here's an example of what a new graduate's profile might look like:

> Resourceful Registered Nurse with healthcare experience as a Certified Emergency Medical Technician and a proven work history, ready to apply transferable skills, including first-aid and basic life support, and a lifelong interest in nursing. Excels in settings requiring independent decision-making as well as team collaboration. Excellent organizational and critical thinking skills.

This is what a more experienced nurse might write:

> Highly motivated and resourceful Registered Nurse with demonstrated effectiveness in the managed care environment as well as solid medical-surgical experience in acute care and community settings. Proficient in communicating and facilitating the acceptance of controversial managed-care concepts. Excels in advocating for patients within this cost-sensitive environment. Capable of prioritizing multiple responsibilities in fast-paced environments.

3. Your Education and Credentials

If this section becomes too lengthy, consider including a portion of it after the description of your professional experience.

License and Certification

Identify the state(s) in which you are licensed. It is not necessary to include your license number. Instead, carry your license in your professional portfolio, described below, and take it with you to the interview. Include professional board certification from the American Nurses Credentialing Center (ANCC) and other professional associations.

Education

Place in reverse chronological order, including if currently enrolled. This section is for your formal nursing education, undergraduate and graduate.

Continuing Education

An extremely important "selling" and balancing feature to compensate for gaps or deficiencies in formal education or experience.

Professional Affiliations and Membership

Another important "selling" and balancing feature.

Special Abilities

Such as foreign languages spoken, sign language, and computer skills (highly recommended!)

Awards and Honors

This is no time for modesty. If you've won any, say so.

Publications and Presentations

Mention any articles you may have written or any occasion where you were required to convey educational information to groups of people.

Examples of how this might look are:

License and Certification	• Registered Professional Nurse, New York and New Jersey • Certified Medical-Surgical Nurse, ANCC
Education	• Bachelor of Science, Nursing, Adelphi University (in progress) • A.A.S., Nursing, Elmont School of Nursing, New York, NY (1992)
Continuing Education	• Basic Cardiac Life Support • AACN Cardiology Education Update '98 • Case Management for staff nurses • IV Certification
Professional Affiliations	• American Association of Critical Care Nurses • Sigma Theta Tau International Nursing Honor Society • New York State Nurses Association
Special Abilities	• Fluent in Spanish and sign language • Beginning competence with computers, including Windows, word processing, and the Internet.
Awards and Honors	• Dean's List, Salem Community College (1990) • Outstanding Academic Achievement Award, Salem Community College (1988) • Listed in *Who's Who Among American College Students* (1992) • Distinguished Nursing Practice Award, Circle Hospital Center (1991)
Publications and Presentations	• *Care of the Dying Patient Brooklyn Hospital* (1989) • Mentoring of New Graduates, Brooklyn Hospital (1991) • "Transition to home care for acute care nurses," *Nursing Management* (1996)

4. Description of Your Experience

List your relevant jobs in reverse chronological order (meaning, your most recent experience appears first) in any of the following categories that apply:

- **Professional nursing experience:** For work as an R.N. or nursing student
- **Additional healthcare experience:** For jobs other than R.N.; such as LPN, nursing assistant, and emergency medical technician
- **Additional work experience:** For work outside of healthcare
- **Volunteer work experience:** for unpaid experiences (highly recommended!)

Use action verbs such as *provided, taught, created,* and *supervised* in your descriptions (see list below). When describing work experiences outside of healthcare, identify and describe relevant transferable skills. Examples of a transferable skills are: triage of accident victims as an emergency medical technician, or customer-service skills used when employed as a bank teller.

Management and Leadership Skills

administered	coordinated	delegated	improved	planned
supervised	developed	assigned	directed	initiated
produced	led	established	managed	scheduled
organized	headed			

Communication and People Skills

conferred	interacted	referred	interacted	participated
explained	clarified	lectured	collaborated	defined
formulated	listened	communicated	described	developed
directed	consulted			

Research Skills

analyzed	clarified	researched	collected	formulated
compared	gathered	searched	conducted	identified
critiqued	detected	determined	interviewed	diagnosed
evaluated	investigated	located	organized	

Technical Skills

adapted	applied	developed	replaced	maintained
solved	specialized	converted	studied	utilized
designed	determined	remodeled	restored	

Teaching Skills

adapted	developed	individualized	taught	clarified
encouraged	coached	evaluated	instructed	trained
motivated	transmitted	conducted	facilitated	coordinated

Financial and Data Skills

administered	projected	forecasted	managed	appraised
measured	assessed	planned	prepared	developed

Creative Skills

designed	adapted	originated	began	performed
initiated	composed	conceptualized	revitalized	created
reshaped				

Helping Skills

adapted	coached	advocated	collaborated	contributed
rehabilitated	assessed	assisted	diagnosed	helped
cared for	educated			

Organization and Detail Skills

complied	organized	reviewed	prepared	processed
scheduled	distributed	maintained	provided	charted
executed	monitored	generated	collected	implemented
ordered				

Verbs for Additional Accomplishments

achieved	pioneered	completed	expanded	resolved
transformed	restored	improved		

To create phrases for your résumé, begin each entry with an action verb, and write the phrase "telegram style" rather than in full sentences, as suggested in the book *Résumés, Résumés, Résumés* (Career Press, 1995). The list of action verbs that follow (adapted from Yana Parker's *Résumé Pro*) is divided into categories of job skills relevant to the descriptions you might be creating.

Each description should include dates of employment, job title, name and address of organization (city and state are sufficient, full address can appear on application, if necessary). Start each description of your work experience with a phrase that orients the reader to the size and nature of the agency for whom you worked, as well as the general scope of your responsibilities. Following this orienting phrase, create additional short and pithy phrases that describe your most important responsibilities and achievements. Avoid repetition if similar responsibilities occurred in more than one job.

Examples are:

1990 to present	*Clinical Office Coordinator, Bronx Oncology Associates, Bronx, NY*

- Provide nursing care and administrative support to a high volume, 19 R.N., 8 M.D. practice for the diagnosis and cutting-edge treatment of cancer.

- Perform telephone triage, including intervention and referral.

- Conduct independent nursing assessments and develop plans of care in collaboration with physicians.

- Provide education, counseling and emotional support to patients and families.

- Act as liaison between patient, physicians, and health care institutions.

- Coordinate inpatient, outpatient and office services, including the monitoring of plans of care to ensure compliance with insurance reimbursement policies.

1992 to 1994	*Student Clinical Rotations, St. Joseph's School of Nursing, Staten Island, NY*

- Learned and practiced primary nursing care in collaboration with professional nursing staff and multidisciplinary team in a variety of clinical settings, including Med-Surg, ICU, CCU, ER, Pediatrics, Maternity, and Psychiatry.

- Developed, implemented and revised written nursing care plans, including discharge planning

- Provided teaching and emotional support to patients and families.

1988 to 1990   *Emergency Medical Technician, Brooklyn Emergency Medical Services, Brooklyn, NY*

- Provided pre-hospital emergency care, for sick and injured patients as part of a two-person ambulance response team.

- Provided intervention at the scene, including triage, treatment, transport to treating facility and status report to receiving staff.

- Initiated and maintained advanced cardiac life support, including defibrilation at scene and during transport.

- Acted as preceptor to newly hired Emergency Medical Technicians.

1992 to 1994   *Staff Nurse, Mount Olive Medical Center, New York, NY*

- Provided primary nursing care to adults with complex medical-surgical illnesses, often requiring critical care interventions on a 40-bed unit specializing in oncology, pain management, and hematological disorders.

- Proficient in a broad range of critical care skills such as hemodynamic monitoring, ventilator care, titration of cardiac medications, and advanced life support.

- Responsible for written nursing care plans, including assessment and intervention of rapidly changing patient status.

- Assigned to frequent charge responsibilities.

A completed résumé might look like this:

SALLY SMITH, B.S.N., R.N.
75 East Main Street, #7A
New York, NY 10010
(212) 555-9831

Profile
Highly motivated and resourceful Registered Nurse with current experience and a proven track record in providing nursing care for the stable and critically ill adult and geriatric patient. Capable of managing multiple assignments simultaneously and efficiently. Excels in environments requiring independent decision-making and team collaboration. Able to interact effectively with management, staff, and patients from all levels and cultural backgrounds.

License
- Registered Professional Nurse, New York State License

Education
- Bachelor of Science, Nursing, The City College of New York, New York, NY (1986)

Continuing Education
- Basic CPR Certification
- EKG and Cardiac Arrhythmias (1998)
- IV Certification
- Basic computer keyboard and Internet skills
- HIV Nursing Care Strategies

Awards
- 1992 Nursing Employee of the Year, Oceanside Medical Center, NewYork, NY

Professional Membership
- American Nurses Association, member
- New York State Nurses Association, member

Additional Abilities
- Fluent in Spanish and Sign Language
- Computer competence, including Windows, word processing, and the Internet.

Professional Experience

1994 to present   *Staff Nurse, Radiology Department, Mount Olive Medical Center, New York, NY.*

- Provide primary nursing care during a broad range of radiologic procedures to in-patients and out-patients of all ages with medical-surgical problems.

Sally Smith, page 2

- Manage the nursing care needs of stable as well as critically ill patients during and while awaiting procedures.

- Assist during complex procedures such as MRIs and angiographies, including pre- and post-procedure assessment, and support of patient well-being during procedure.

- Administer oral contrast material; insert and monitor IV during administration of IV contrast.

- Assess and manage allergic and life-threatening responses to procedures.

- Provide patient and family teaching, including emotional support.

- Participate in quality assurance activities, including patient surveys and documentation.

1989 to 1994   *Staff Nurse, Intensive Care Unit, Oceanside Hospital, New York, NY.*

- Provided primary nursing care to adult and geriatric high risk patients with complex medical and surgical needs on six-bed ICUs with a ratio of 1 R.N. to 2–3 patients.

- Responsible for written nursing care plans which included assessment and intervention of rapidly changing patient status, in collaboration with multi-disciplinary team.

- Performed a broad range of critical care skills, including hemodynamic monitoring for patients with multisystem failure.

- Assigned to frequent charge responsibilities.

1986 to 1989   *Staff Nurse, Medicine, Highview Hospital, New York, NY.*

- Provided primary nursing care to adult and geriatric patients with medical and neurological problems on a 26-bed acute care unit.

- Responsibilities included nursing care plans, including discharge planning; patient and family education, including emotional support; multidisciplinary collaboration.

- Assigned to frequent charge responsibilities.

Cover letters

A cover letter needs to accompany the résumé you give to prospective employers. A different cover letter should be written for each employment situation, rather than using a general letter to cover all circumstances. Once you customize one cover letter, it can be used as a kind of template, a model from which to create others. Yana Parker, in her book, *The Résumé Pro*, suggests you think about the following questions to help you prepare your letter:

- Why do you want to work for that organization?
- What do you know about the organization?
- How did you hear about them?
- What do you know about the position you are applying for?
- How can you help that organization with its goals, i.e., what skills, competencies, and abilities do you have to offer?

Guidelines for a good cover letter, adapted from recommendations made by Parker, include:

- Address your letter to the person with the authority to hire you, or who has been designated to interview you for the position, i.e., the Nurse Recruiter or other administrator. When unable to obtain this information, use a functional title, such as "Dear Nurse Recruiter," not "To whom it may concern," or "Dear Sir or Madam."
- Show that you know a little about the organization.
- Phrase your letter so that it is professional, but still warm and friendly.
- Set yourself apart from the crowd. Try to find at least one thing about you, your skills, competencies, experiences, that is unique, and relevant to the position.
- Be specific. State the position you are applying for, how you heard about the position.
- Be brief, a few short paragraphs, all on one page will suffice.
- Take the initiative about the next step by mentioning what you will do next. For example, "I'll call your office to determine when an interview might be possible." This demonstrates proactivity rather than passivity.

Follow-Up Letters

A follow-up letter is an opportunity to reinforce a positive perception of you. It is a professional way to maintain contact. Because the interview is not unlike a sales experience, the more contact you have with the person contemplating your services, and the more positive a perception they have of you, the more likely it is for you to make the sale, in this case, to land the job. Your follow-up letter should include the following components adapted from Parker's *The Résumé Pro*.

- A statement of appreciation to the interviewer for the opportunity to discuss the job opportunity
- A reference, to something that was discussed, as a reminder and reinforcement of your experience, skills, etcetera
- Additional information, or new reasons that you are interested in the job, perhaps based on what was discovered or exchanged in the interview
- An offer to provide additional information or participate in additional interviews conducted by others
- A clarification, when necessary, about something that was discussed in the interview, such as a question that was asked or an issue to which you want to add information
- An anticipation of hearing from them again, perhaps about a favorable outcome, or at least about the decision that will be made

Business Cards

Business cards are a relatively easy and inexpensive sales tool to produce and create that make an impressive professional statement that can set you apart from your competitors. Carry them with you to exchange during seminars and networking events. End an interview with an assertive handshake, a warm smile, and a "leave-behind" in the form of a business card. Attach them to your résumé to circulate at job fairs.

Create a Professional Portfolio

A professional portfolio is a representative sample, a collection of documents about who you are professionally and what you have to offer. It contains an accumulation of information related to your professional life; a kind of historical chronology of your activities. It's almost a kind of professional diary. It contains the documented elements and examples, such as copies of your credentials, diplomas, letters of reference and recommendation, of your professional identity, gathered into one portable package that can be carried to interviews.

Your portfolio can have a private and a public section. The private section can be used to safeguard and keep track of important professional documents, accounts of your nursing worklife, such as your license, certification information, and continuing education dates. You select from the private section of your portfolio what would be most relevant at a job interview. The public section is what you want others to see about you and what you have to offer. It's a sales tool, like a marketing book used by salespeople to demonstrate their wares. It may be tailored for the occasion by supplementing it with material from the private section of your portfolio, as indicated.

In her book, *Networking for Career Advancement*, Valarie Restifo recommends including the following in your portfolio:

- Broadcast letter that introduces you
- Letters of recommendation
- Typed list of three to six personal and professional references
- Published articles or other samples of your work, as described above
- Business cards
- Your résumé

Many nurses have long used a variation of this portfolio as a filing system to keep these professional documents safe, as well as accessible when needed. Today's business-savvy nurse takes this a step further and uses her portfolio as a sales tool, as a way to stand out from others. In addition, because 21st century nurses will be moving around the healthcare workplace much more frequently than those in previous generations, your portfolio becomes an important traveling companion to chronicle your travels and keep the historical data about it organized. In some ways it may serve as a way to reminisce and recount, and then to feel proud about where you've been and what you've done. It can become the mobile equivalent of your own personnel file, similar to the one your employer keeps about you, serving to remind you of your accomplishments.

Your portfolio can be as creative and imaginative as you are and, in fact, is an actual demonstration to a potential employer about your creativity, confidence, and assertiveness. It becomes a selling feature in and of itself! Consider using a colorful binder with interesting dividers. Take care, however, that it doesn't get too information-intensive, complex, or overdone; keep it unique and professional.

While a résumé can convey only an overview of what you have done, a portfolio is a way to supplement this and actually demonstrate what the résumé can only describe. In this way, your portfolio becomes another sales tool. Bring it to the interview with you so that you can show as well as tell! Your portfolio should include:

- Résumé
- Letters of reference
- Names and addresses of people providing references and recommendations
- Letters of recommendation
- Professional credentials, including diplomas, transcripts, continuing education and contact hour certificates
- Samples of professional activities, including performance appraisals, letters of commendation or recognition, representations of articles you have published, presentations you have given, poster sessions you have done, and anything that documents a value-added activity

Chapter 12

Selling Your Skills

An interview is a sales experience in which the potential employer is your customer. In fact, all of the healthcare marketplace contains potential customers to whom you can consider selling your services. This can be an especially optimistic way to frame your career security in a growth industry with ever-multiplying matches between your nursing skills and competencies and the marketplace needs. The interview is an opportunity for you to present your best features translated into your credentials, experience, talents, and skills, to the potential employers. You must convince them, sell them on the idea that you have what they need, and that they should "buy" what you have to offer, namely your capacity not only to do the job that needs to be done, but to excel at it. Convincing them that you can do more than the status quo is what can separate you from the competition, from the many others with the same qualifications. Take the situation of Millie, a newly graduated nurse who is composing a follow-up letter to the interview she just had. The nurse manager told her that they expect 100 percent from their employees, so she wrote the following in her letter: "You said that you expected 100 percent from your staff, and I wanted you to know that you can count on 120 percent from me." Millie was making an attempt to convince—or sell—the nurse manager that she would go beyond the expected. By the way, she got the job!

Richard Bolles, author of *What Color is Your Parachute?*, describes the interview as the occasion on which you "show the person who has the power to hire you how your

> "You are living juicy! Ride into your life on a creative cycle, full of juice, abundance, and ecstatic wonderment. You are a star."
>
> —Sark, *Living Juicy*

skills can help them with their problems." This will require several things from you. First, you need a thorough knowledge of your transferable and marketable skills and your qualifications, translated into and matched for what the current marketplace needs. Anticipate some degree of change in the marketplace every six months requiring a retooling of your skills. You have had an opportunity to explore how to improve the marketability of your skills in chapter 8, "Marketplace Research." Second, you need knowledge of the potential employer's problems; what job needs to be done and what's different about this organization's needs that you are qualified to take care of. And third, you need to conceptualize the interview as a sales experience so that you can convince—or, again, sell—the employer that you are the best person for the job that needs to be done. Test your interview knowledge below:

THE INTERVIEW: TRUE OR FALSE?

1. In order to appear natural and spontaneous, it is better *not* to prepare responses ahead of time. True or false?

2. Be cautious about your body language because *40–50 percent* of communication is nonverbal. True or false?

3. It is important to maintain direct eye contact at all times with the interviewer.

4. It is better to interrupt the interviewer than to forget to say or ask something.

5. Referring to a list when asking questions gives the impression of being unprepared. True or false?

6. Asking for a tour of the unit appears intrusive.

7. Asking about the next steps or what your chances are of getting the job is too aggressive. True or false? True or false?

8. Writing a follow-up letter to the interview is redundant and a waste of the interviewer's time as well as yours. True or false?

9. If you decide to take another position before you hear the results of the interview, it's better to withdraw your application without saying why. True or false?

10. If you do not get the job, it is not a good idea to discuss the reasons why with the interviewer. True or false?

ANSWERS

1. False. Preparation is essential for successful interviewing. It also helps you to lower your anxiety and manage your stress.

2. False! A whopping 90 to 95 percent of communication is nonverbal and takes the form of body language, manner of dress, tone of voice, attitude, and behaviors such as punctuality, assertiveness, etcetera.

3. False. No one maintains eye contact 100 percent of the time. Looking away periodically and briefly as you ponder the answers to questions is normal.

4. False. A better option is to jot down notes about questions you have and wait for the best opportunity to ask them, perhaps at the end of the interview, or when asked if you have questions. However, flexibility is the key here. If you are confused, it's better to clarify this with a polite interruption rather than feel lost and unable to respond or continue.

5. False. Just the opposite is true. Bringing a list makes you look prepared and interested enough to have given considered thought to the employment situation. It will also decrease your anxiety.

6. False. This is an appropriate request. Taking a tour can provide a different and perhaps welcome source of data that words cannot completely convey.

7. False. This is an assertive question that conveys confidence and professionalism. It is also an essential sales strategy for planning your follow-up and the focus of your efforts and energy. Assertiveness and productivity are essential characteristics of successful 21st century nurses, and well worth strengthening your skills in.

8. False. Not only does this kind of follow-up demonstrate that you know how to conduct yourself professionally, it also continues contact with the employer beyond the interview to keep your name familiar. In addition, it gives you the opportunity to strengthen weak responses caused by anxiety or insufficient preparation.

9. False. A written letter expressing appreciation for the time and consideration granted you and a brief reason for your decision maintains the relationship and keeps the door open for future possibilities. It is also a way to grow your network as well as your reputation.

10. False. Asking this question could strengthen your approach for the next interview and may also keep the door open for the future should another job at that organization become available.

The Interview as a Sales Experience

If the image of a pushy used car salesman or intrusive telemarketer comes into your head when you think about selling, let's discuss a less stereotypical way to think about selling so that you can benefit from this extremely important and useful career strategy. Believe it or not, you already are a salesperson!

Sales is a natural part of all communication; in fact, sales is inherent in almost all conversation. Every time you talk to someone about your point of view, every time you attempt to convince another person to do something they may feel unsure of, an element of sales in involved. In fact, right now I am a salesperson trying to "sell" you on the idea that sales is something that you can do, should do, and actually already do. I want you to "buy" this concept. And right now, you are a salesperson too! You may be trying to sell me or someone with whom you may discuss this concept that sales can never be a part of your life as a nurse, or that it is incompatible with the caring and nurturing component of nursing. Nothing can be farther from the truth.

Teaching a new diabetic to perform the insulin injections she is convinced she cannot do is a sales experience. Or, reassuring a new mother that she will indeed learn how to care for her first newborn is also a kind of selling. As is teaching sex education to an adolescent and explaining the need for protected sex. The same element of persuasive salesmanship that is involved in patient education can be used on your own behalf in a job interview. In fact, in a competitive marketplace, it is what can make the difference between you and others with the same credentials and experience. Just as a sales person can be a helpful ally in your quest for purchasing something you need but may not completely understand, so can you be helpful to both the employer and yourself in your mutual quest for a satisfying and productive employment relationship.

Preparation for the Interview

At least 50 percent of the interview takes place before you walk in the door. More accurately put, the interview process begins with the very first contact you have with the potential employer, whether it's the impression your cover letter and résumé makes, how you conduct yourself in a spontaneous interview at a job fair, or how you interact with a receptionist on the phone. A good salesperson would not miss these opportunities to "close the deal." In fact, in sales there are a series of "closes" required before the actual sale, the final "close," occurs; for example, a job interview is only the first "close" to finish before the hiring process is complete.

Closes are like stages and each one is a minisuccess on the way to getting the job offer, the final "close." A first close is what you have to do to get the interview. This could include your cover letter, your résumé/advertisement, and the follow-up letter you send. A salesperson doesn't just ask you if you want to buy something; he might also show it to you, ask if he can keep in touch, send free samples, ask when he can meet with you. And this is what you can do as well. One of the biggest mistakes nurses make with regard to this first close is their reluctance to do the follow-up essential to keeping the potential employer's attention. This is partly related to the influence of the pushy salesman stereotype, and partly about lack of knowledge since the application of these business strategies is a relatively new concept applied to nursing careers. Other factors that require attention on your part are difficulty with assertiveness or the fear of rejection.

Continuing with the analogy of the salesperson, many sales books and seminars are devoted to helping salespeople overcome this problem. The message of these books can be boiled down to the following facts:

1. Not everyone will be interested in your product or service.

2. A percentage of people *will* buy it, perhaps 10 percent (one in 10).

3. This percentage can sometimes fluctuate to a higher percentage depending on marketplace issues such as increased or decreased needs.

4. If one in 10 (10 percent) of the people will buy, that means that it may take nine "no's" to get to the one "yes"

5. In a competitive market, the more "no's" you get, the closer you are to the eventual "yes," as long as you don't abort the process and give up trying.

6. Even if someone is interested, that does not mean he will buy it at that time.

7. Because the potential to buy at a later date exists, staying in touch is essential to this future prospect and to building your network.

8. These and other factors, may contribute to objections the employer has to buying your "services."

9. Your challenge is to do the best you can to overcome potential objections and close the deal or land the job.

Understanding these facts can take the sting out of rejection and place it in the statistical and nonpersonal frame of reference, where it belongs. These facts also form the basis for the sales skills you need in the interview process. They become the guidelines upon which to build a successful strategy.

Preparation for the interview also involves anticipating questions you will be asked and developing responses for them. This kind of anticipatory preparation can help you control your anxiety. Keep in mind that anxiety in its mild state is actually motivating since the adrenaline that naturally accompanies will keep you alert, sharp, and able to meet unexpected challenges that may arise in the interview. Moderate or severe anxiety can prevent you from doing your best and eventually affect your confidence and self-esteem. If the strategies described in this section do not ease your anxiety sufficiently, it may be helpful to work with someone—a mentor, a trusted colleague, or perhaps, a coach—so that personalized attention can address your particular concern.

Tips for Managing Your Anxiety

Job interviews make everyone at least a little nervous. Here are some tips for managing your anxiety:

Arrive Early

Be compulsive about this. Consider arriving at least one hour prior to the time of the interview. Giving yourself this extra hour allows for unexpected travel delays (which can escalate your anxiety wildly) as well as difficulty in finding the interview location. Upon arrival, go directly to the place of the interview so that you know exactly where it is, and then leave until it is time for the interview. Go to a place where you can sit quietly, grounding and centering yourself, using a relaxation strategy that works best for you, perhaps by deep breathing or meditation. Try sitting in a quiet place of worship, going to a coffee shop and having a decaffeinated beverage, walking in a nearby park, or just wandering around the block a few times. Use the same preparation principle as when you study for exams: At some point prior to the exam, let go and stop studying. Clear your head. Say a prayer if that helps. Let go and trust that the information you need will be there when needed, emerging spontaneously when you have prepared effectively.

Carry a Briefcase

A briefcase or other professional carry-all enhances your image and keeps you organized. It can contain your professional portfolio along with additional copies of your résumé, other show-and-tell documents, and examples of your accomplishments. Also bring paper and pen, a list of previously prepared questions that you want to ask, and any other notes of reminder to yourself. You may even want to carry an inspirational quote or a prayer if this kind of strategy helps you to feel calm. The extra copies of your résumé can be given to the interviewer should yours not be available for some unforeseen reason, or to additional people who might interview you. You can refer to your own résumé as you respond to questions, especially about such information as dates of employment. Rather than interrupt the interviewer with questions, jot down brief notes while the interviewer is talking and ask them at the end of the interview or at a time that seems appropriate.

Use the Follow-Up Letter to Strengthen "Weak" Responses

Your anxiety will be minimized if you know that you can add information you might have forgotten or even provide a stronger response to a question you believe you didn't handle well. An effective way to do this is to include a brief explanation along with your "improved" response in the follow-up letter (which needs to be sent whether or not this remedy is needed, and will be discussed below). Here's how it can work:

Iris Carter, a new B.S.N. graduate, prepared for what she heard (through networking and informational interviewing) could be a very tough interview at a large New York City teaching hospital where she had her heart set on working. She knew that she would be given a patient care scenario and asked to discuss how she would care for the patient. The scenario she was given was the following: "You are the nurse in the PACU and a patient who just had an abdominal hysterectomy is wheeled in from the OR. Give me two nursing diagnoses and two interventions for this patient." How prepared might you be to answer such a question? What would your answer be? More seasoned nurses could be asked some variation of this question related to work experiences they have had.

The diagnoses provided by Iris in response to the question were related to the potential for bleeding and the potential for airway obstruction. After Iris offered several interventions for each, she felt satisfied with her response. As she reflected on the interview later, she realized that she had forgotten an extremely important intervention, namely that she would monitor the patient's dressing for bleeding. Her initial panic subsided when she realized that she could use the follow-up letter she would be writing to remedy the situation. At first she considered ignoring the situation altogether, hoping the interviewer hadn't noticed or in some way that it would not matter. She rejected this idea as wishful thinking and rightly decided that it may do more harm than good to ignore it. She included the following paragraph in her letter:

> In thinking back to the question you asked about the patient with the abdominal hysterectomy, I realized I neglected to tell you that I would check the dressing for bleeding. This is something I would know to do but didn't tell you because I was a bit anxious in the interview. If you would like to know anything more about my ability to care for this kind of patient, please let me know. As we discussed in the interview, my medical-surgical clinical rotations included the care of many newly post-operative patients, and I have confidence in my ability to care for them effectively.

This explanation says a lot about Iris's integrity and professionalism, as well as her salesmanship. She comes across as someone who can recognize and remedy human failings that can affect quality patient care, a very strong selling feature indeed. She is also demonstrating assertiveness in her communication and confidence in herself, in her ability to do the job, and in her ability to solve the employer's problems. It is unclear whether or not the interviewer was already satisfied with her initial response. Perhaps she was, making this response unnecessary. What is clear, however, is how Iris took charge of the situation and how she was able to compensate for the anxiety she felt in the interview.

Preparing Responses

What you are asked depends on the skill of the interviewer, who may be just as uncomfortable about this experience as you. What follows are samples of questions you may be asked, along with weak responses to avoid and stronger responses that sell or convince more effectively. Note that the responses are ideal, and may sound a bit stiff or academic to you. Since it is unlikely that you will be asked all of them, use them as a guide to prepare your own responses. You might also use these questions as a kind of self-assessment, preparing responses for all of them to give you a clearer picture of yourself as a nurse, perhaps indicating areas needing more attention or pointing to areas of strength.

Anticipated question:	Why do you want to work here?
Ineffective response:	You have good benefits.
Effective Response:	You have an excellent reputation for patient care, and I am ready for the challenges of a tertiary care medical center.
Anticipated question:	What makes you qualified to work on this kind of neurology unit?
Ineffective response:	I'm a hard worker.
Effective Response:	In my med-surg and community health rotations, I cared for a number of neuro patients. I realized I was good at the complexity of it. In addition, I've recently completed a continuing education course on the physical assessment of the neuro patient.
Anticipated question:	What are your strengths?
Ineffective response:	I like people and people like me.
Effective response:	I'm flexible and able to adapt quickly. I'm also a good organizer, and work well with others.
Anticipated question:	What continuing education have you recently participated in?
Ineffective response:	A lot of different courses. Sometimes I send in those AJN tests; you know, those articles.
Effective response:	I've just completed ACLS. I'm presently enrolled in peripheral and central IV certification. I'm planning to take an advanced physical assessment course in two months.

Anticipated question:	Tell me about your experience.
Ineffective response:	I've had experience in a lot of different areas, as you can see on my résumé. (Note: Yes, the interviewers can read your résumé. However, they also want to hear you talk about it, so this is an opportunity. A good résumé should inspire questions in the interviewers' minds, giving you an opportunity to add to it, clarify, and shape a response to the job you are selling your services for.)
Effective response:	While I don't yet have R.N. experience, I have three years of hospital-related experience as a unit clerk and nursing assistant. My clinical rotations provided experience in all aspects of nursing, especially neuro patients, since we did our med-surg rotation on neuro.
Anticipated question:	What do you want from this experience?
Ineffective response:	I want to work days and I need health insurance.
Effective response:	An opportunity to develop professionally, to share my ideas and skills. I am seeking new professional challenges. I also want to use this experience to qualify for ANCC board certification in med-surg nursing.
Anticipated question:	Why did you choose to become a nurse?
Ineffective response:	I like to help people.
Effective response:	It's a profession that offers upward mobility, diverse challenges, and the kind of personal contact I've always enjoyed.
Anticipated question:	Tell me what you like to do best in nursing.
Ineffective answer:	Making people feel better.
Effective answer:	I'm a good teacher, especially when it involves something complex like insulin administration. I know how to explain complicated things simply and it's gratifying to experience people's response to it.
Anticipated question:	How do you deal with conflicts on the job?
Ineffective answer:	I never have conflicts. I get along with everyone.
Effective answer:	I suggest that we discuss the issue to clarify the problem and check for misinterpretations. Conflicts are a natural part of the job and communication is essential to working them out.

Anticipated question:	If I were to call your former employer for a reference, what would she say about you?
Ineffective answer:	She would say I'm a good worker.
Effective answer:	I believe she would tell you about my flexibility, especially when the hospital was downsized last year. There was a need for unit clerks to rotate to other units. While I did it to cooperate, I have to say that I gained a lot too. It helped me improve my communication skills since there was more contact with patients and family on the other units.
Anticipated question:	What is your philosophy of nursing?
Ineffective answer:	Never miss a day of work.
Effective answer:	I believe nurses support people for the time that they cannot support themselves, physically, emotionally, or spiritually, always recognizing the point at which they need to be assisted to take over their own care again. Orem's nursing theory of self care most closely matches my ideas about nursing.
Anticipated question:	What are your work-related goals for the next five years?
Ineffective answer:	I don't know. I may be planning a family.
Effective answer:	I would like to be ANCC-certified in med-surg nursing and then begin thinking about graduate school.
Anticipated question:	Why should I hire you instead of other applicants?
Ineffective answer:	I have a lot of experience.
Effective answer:	In addition to my familiarity with the hospital environment because of my work as a unit clerk, I can offer you the same kind of commitment and flexibility that my last employer remarked about in my performance appraisal.
Anticipated question:	Describe yourself.
Ineffective answer:	I'm married, have two children, and work hard.
Effective answer:	I consider myself flexible and enthusiastic. I enjoy the fast-paced nature of the hospital environment. I get along well with people of all backgrounds. I was recently inducted into Sigma Theta Tau, the international nursing honor society.

Anticipated question:	Why did you leave your former job?
Ineffective answer:	I was bored.
Effective answer:	Overall, I liked my last job. However, I felt ready for the challenges of a tertiary care medical center like this one, especially because you specialize in oncology.
Anticipated question:	Since you haven't worked in med-surg for some years, how well will you function here?
Ineffective answer:	Once you've learned med-surg, you never forget it.
Effective answer:	I have recently completed a refresher course. I volunteer at a rehab center regularly. I've also kept up by reading AJN and going to professional conferences. In addition, I'm a fast learner and feel confident in my ability to do this job.
Anticipated question:	Are you IV Certified?
Ineffective answer:	No.
Effective answer:	No. However, I would welcome the opportunity to do this and would become certified if it was a necessary qualification of the job. Also, I have experience in monitoring IV's and managing IV therapy.
Anticipated question:	Have you ever managed a large clinic?
Ineffective answer:	Not really.
Effective answer:	No, but I have successfully managed my brother's graphic design business. Some of my responsibilities were taking telephone orders and resolving customer problems and complaints. I also organized his telephone contacts and developed a filing system of his customers.
Anticipated question:	Have you had experience in home visits?
Ineffective answer:	Yes.
Effective answer:	Yes, during my nursing school clinical rotation. I enjoyed it. I liked the increased autonomy and the more comprehensive assessments that were possible in home environments.

PERSONAL REFLECTION: YOUR PREPARED RESPONSES

To prepare your responses for the interview, review the anticipated questions on the previous pages and then answer the following questions.

1. Reflect on your nursing skills and experience.

Your strengths. This means what you excel at, love doing, and have experience in. This is what you have to sell. Your strengths are:

_____

_____

_____

Your needs and weaknesses. What you are not good at, dislike doing, or have limited or no experience in. These may form the basis of potential objections from the interviewer and you will need to (1) prepare responses designed to overcome the objection, or (2) recognize that this is not a job for which you are well-suited. Your needs and weaknesses are:

_____

_____

_____

2. Reflect on the job for which you are preparing to be interviewed.

What the employer needs is:

_____

_____

_____

What you have to offer or sell (related to the employer's need) is:

_____

_____

_____

Potential objections—concerns that the potential employer might have about your needs or experience that might prevent you from getting a job—are:

_____

_____

_____

3. Identify what you have to do to change a need or weakness identified above into a strength, or at least neutralize it.

_____

_____

_____

_____

4. Develop a prepared response for your needs or weaknesses.

_____

_____

_____

_____

5. Develop a prepared response for your strengths.

_____

_____

_____

_____

6. Develop a prepared response for additional questions you anticipate being asked.

_____

_____

_____

_____

Anticipating Responses to Problem Questions and Special Situations

Injuries or Disabilities

If you have a disability that will prevent you from doing the kind of work you had been able to do prior to being injured, an honest appraisal of what you can now do is essential if you are to convince the employer that you *can* do the job required. For example, if you have always worked on a Med-Surg Unit but a back injury prevents you from the heavy lifting required, you may need to consider working elsewhere, rather than expecting the employer to automatically accommodate you. In the growth industry that healthcare is, there are a multitude of options and opportunities for which your transferable skills can be used. Both you and the employer are better served by an honest analysis of your situation. If you are having trouble selecting an alternative or making the shift, consider talking it over with a mentor a coach.

Termination from a Previous Job

Once again, honesty is the best policy. Because you may feel very sensitive about the situation, preparation will be essential here. Be matter of fact about what happened, do not go into more detail than necessary, but do not avoid it completely or lie about it. Do not blame or criticize the employer who terminated you, and most importantly, focus on the positive, on what you have learned, on what you are able to do now, especially related to the job you are being interviewed for. Some of the preparation for this area may include working on the feelings you have surrounding the termination. If your professional or personal self-esteem is injured, time and reflection—or perhaps professional assistance—may be needed. Keep in mind that being terminated is not necessarily the end of your career and can lead to something quite positive, especially if you move on having learned something you might not have been able to experience otherwise. Remember that Lee Iacocca was fired from Ford Motor Company after decades of loyal service. He went on to a job others didn't want and wound up saving the Chrysler Corporation from bankruptcy.

Gaps in Employment

It is perfectly acceptable not to work consistently all your life. But rather than risk misperceptions about why you didn't work, develop responses that reflect involvement in constructive activities and some transferable skills, like assisting your spouse in a business.

Job Hopping

This term may be obsolete. When once this indicated possible employment instability and restlessness, it now can demonstrate flexibility and the ability to meet new challenges, especially if your prepared responses support this.

Questions You Should Ask

It is likely that you will be given an opportunity to ask questions at some point during the interview. Traditionally, this occurs at the end. The following areas represent some issues you may need to understand, and therefore questions to ask, before making a decision (see the Employer Evaluation Sheet) that a mutually satisfactory match exists between you and the potential employer:

- Role of nurse, including collegial and peer relationships
- Staffing ratios and policies
- In-house education, training, and support, especially for new roles and responsibilities
- Opportunities for and policies about advancement
- The state of organizational restructuring for the job you are being considered for and for the organization in general
- The type of management (hierarchical? team based?), including whom you will be reporting to
- The physical layout. Ask for a tour, if possible
- Salary and benefits

Questions That Should Not Be Asked of You

There are some questions that the law prohibits being asked of you because they are discriminatory and not job related. If you are asked any of these questions, one way to politely refuse to answer is to change the topic, perhaps ask a job-related question. If the interviewer persists (a rare occurrence), you may have to be more direct but nonetheless polite. Also, the presence of these questions may signal a nonmatch between you and the employer since asking these discriminatory questions speak volumes about the organization's corporate culture. These "questionable questions" include your age, marital status, religion, sexual preference, nationality, ethnicity, non-job-related arrests or convictions, and financial status or credit issues.

Additional Tips

Dress for Success

Dress in a conservative manner. For women, this means a tailored suit or simple dress with a below-the-knee length, minimal jewelry, moderate makeup, stockings, low-heeled shoes, and a small handbag to accompany the briefcase in which you carry your professional portfolio. For men, a conservative suit and tie, white shirt, polished shoes, and your portfolio. Both women and men should omit perfume or cologne or at least keep it minimal.

Keep Your Answers Brief

Be as direct and succinct as possible. Find the balance between offering too much or too little. One-word answers don't give you the opportunity to "sell." Offering too much information, especially if it's not related to the question, can take both of you off track.

Don't Attempt to Memorize Your Responses

Use your prepared responses as rehearsal tools prior to the interview and then let go of them. They will be stored in your subconscious mind until you need them.

Use Visualization to Enhance Your Memory and Relax Yourself Prior to the Interview

Visualization is another kind of thinking, a state of mind in which attention is focused inward on mental impressions, images, and sensations for the purpose of relaxation or, in this case, problem-solving. Visualization is said to create biochemical and cellular changes as the autonomic nervous system responds to mental imagery. For example, with practice, it is possible to experience a warming of parts of your body even though you are cold by visualizing yourself warmed by the sun. Yvonne Vissing (AJN, 1991) described how "visualization becomes real when the idea of 'creating one's own reality' through use of imagination becomes experience rather than theory." She conducted a study in which nurses who were having interpersonal difficulties on an patient care unit were divided into two groups. One group was taught standard communication skills and conflict resolution. The other group was taught the same content but in addition they were taught how to visualize a positive outcome to the situation. A direct relationship was found between the amount of time spent visualizing and the effects that were experienced. "The individuals who spent the most time visualizing experienced the greatest actual effects." To apply these findings to your interview situation, spend part of your preparation time seeing the outcome as you want it to be, imagining the employer offering you the job, and visualizing yourself answering even the most difficult or unexpected questions confidently and assertively. Consider the words of the *Bhagavad-Gita*: "Man is made by his belief. As he believes, so he is."

Use Affirmations to Enhance your Self-Talk and Increase Your Confidence

An affirmation is a statement you make to yourself that emphasizes your intention and expectation for a positive outcome to a situation. If your thoughts (represented by your self-talk) are hopeful and optimistic, then you will respond with equally hopeful and optimistic actions. Likewise, when negative thoughts and feelings predominate, behaviors and actions tend to be hopeless and pessimistic. Barbara Dossey, author of *Holistic Nursing*, describes the relationship between affirmations and body responses as follows: "When negative thoughts and emotions dominate, the body responds with tightness, uneasiness, an increase in respirations, blood pressure and heart rate, just to name a few physiological responses." This uneasiness will increase the mild anxiety that frequently accompanies interviews and send it soaring into less manageable levels. Affirmations are a way to lessen this anxiety and, when used frequently and regularly, can even help to alter long-held perceptions and beliefs that prevent the growth and risk taking essential to 21st century career management. For additional information about the power of affirmations, see the appendix. Examples of affirmations you can use to strengthen your interviewing ability include:

- I can interview successfully
- I can recall my prepared responses in a spontaneous way
- I am confident about my sales ability
- I can convince the employer that I am the best person for this job
- I have excellent experience and credentials

Hint: for a powerful self-management strategy, use both affirmations and visualization!

Learn about the Organization

The more you know, the better your prepared responses will be, the more professional you will appear, and the more data you will have to make your decision. Ways to learn about the organization include informational interviewing (see below), searching the Internet, reading published reports, and scanning newspaper articles.

Conduct Informational Interviews

An informational interview is a formal discussion you have with someone who knows about the job or the organization you are considering. It's a way to get the inside scoop on the situation. You can formalize a potentially informal chat by setting up an appointment, taking the person to lunch or buying them coffee, and telling them the purpose of the meeting so that they have time to consider helpful responses for you. Informally catching someone on the run who may not have had time to think about the situation may not result in effective data. Consider preparing a list of questions that include:

- Do you like your work? Is it what you expected?
- What is the communication and relationship like between staff and management?
- What is a typical day like for you?

> "I beg you to have patience with everything unresolved in your heart and try to love the questions themselves as if they were locked rooms or books written in a very foreign language. . . . Perhaps then, someday far in the future, you will gradually, without even noticing it, live your way to the answer."
>
> —Rainer Maria Rilke, *Letters to a Young Poet*

• How are disputes and conflicts handled?

• What advice would you give to someone considering working here?

Find the Mutual Match Between Your Strengths and the Employer's Needs

Pursuing or accepting a job where this match does not exist is a waste of time and effort for both you and the employer. Remember that you are interviewing your potential employer just as much as they are interviewing you. Think of the interview as the data collection and assessment part of the nursing process you've learned to apply to patient care, now applied to you.

Use the following Employer Evaluation Sheet to help you decide if a mutually satisfying match exists. Make a photocopy of this sheet for every employer that you interview with and use it to help you rate, keep track of, and compare the data from each interview. Score each statement according to the scale at the top, and then add up the scores to get each organization's total. Consider the organization with the highest score most seriously. Note: Some of these answers may be best obtained through informational interviewing. An additional method of decision making is listing the pros and cons of each situation you are considering. This is best done over a period of time—even a few days—rather than in one sitting.

EMPLOYER EVALUATION SHEET

Score   0 = Unsatisfactory or missing data
            1 = Fair
            2 = Good
            3 = Excellent

_____ The institution bases its policies and procedures on specified standards of nursing practice.

_____ You will be reporting to a nursing administrator as opposed to a non-nursing administrator. (In general, it is better to be reporting to a nursing administrator, however, in the team-based environments arising today, this leadership may vary).

_____ The roles and responsibilities for the nursing position were explained clearly and adequately. _Score an extra point if the description was given in writing._

_____ The nurse-patient ratio was described and is reasonable. _Score an extra point if there is an approved administrative mechanism to negotiate a potentially unreasonable assignment (often called "protest of assignment")_

_____ There are opportunities for administrative and/or clinical advancement.

_____ The orientation for newly hired staff sounds adequate. _Score an extra point for a preceptor program._

_____ There is continuing education and on-site training, especially for new roles and responsibilities. _Score an extra point if off-site training and education is encouraged, and an additional point is some remuneration is provided._

_____ The starting salary for the position is satisfactory.

_____ The benefits package (health/life/disability insurance, vacations, holidays) is satisfactory.

Specify additional factors to be considered on the following lines and score as above:

_____   _____

_____   _____

Chapter 13

Continuing the Journey

Life is a journey, not a destination. And your nursing career can be one of the more interesting journeys you can have along the pathways of your life. What an exciting time to be a nurse! This is a time when oceans of possibilities await those willing to take charge of their nursing destinies by learning to:

- Navigate the white waters of change
- Imitate flexible willow trees rather than rigid oaks
- See the glass as at least half filled rather than half empty

I hope what you read in this book has strengthened you for your journey and assists you to imagine the possible, remember your power, and transcend disillusionment. For the times of doubt and discouragement that are part of all journeys worth taking, I give you the story of Tillie the Turtle. May the memory of her experience strengthen you for the worthwhile challenges ahead.

The Adventure of Tillie the Turtle

Once there was a turtle named Tillie who lived on a tiny island not much bigger than she was. Tillie was a land turtle, not a sea turtle, and while she loved looking at all the water surrounding her, she never went in it much. Oh, sometimes she'd stick a flipper in the water, but swim in it? No. Stories about swift, dangerous currents and sharks kept her on her safe island.

One day she noticed that the water level was rising at the shore. On each succeeding day after that, the tide came in earlier and the water rose higher until it seemed obvious that the island was sinking and soon would be under water. What would she do?

She looked around and saw many of her turtle friends in panic, tool. Some pulled back into their shells, while others peeked out in fear and disbelief. She also saw some of her friends swimming and wondered how they did that. After all, weren't they land turtles like her?

Soon there was no time left to ponder. The water had almost completely submerged the island and was rising to submerge her as well. Convinced she would sink, she felt herself carried off by the motion of the water. "The currents are here at last!" she cried. "I'm done for!"

She thrashed her flippers in fear, convinced she was sinking, not swimming. Soon she realized the thrashing motion was becoming more of a rhythmic motion that was actually propelling her in the water. Soon she relaxed a bit, and the thrashing became even more rhythmic and her powerful flippers seemed to know what to do without her thinking too much about it. She was swimming. Maybe she was a combination of both land and sea turtle.

Soon she looked back. Her island was gone, and there was water all around her. Yes, there were currents, one of her greatest fears, but they were actually helpful when she let them carry her along. And, when the currents were going in a direction she didn't want, her tail made a perfect rudder to steer her in the direction she preferred. When she saw sharks, she just retreated into her strong, protective shell until they got bored and swam away.

She looked around and saw many of her friends smiling back at her, knowingly nodding, each one not sure of where they were going but no longer as worried about the unknown. Somehow the action of swimming was an antidote to the fear they once had. She wondered what would happen next.

It's hard to know what does happen next to Tillie. If you were to continue this story, how would you end it? If you had to write a moral to this story, what might it be? And what will you do when the waters reach *your* shores?

APPENDICES

Appendix A

Resources

Use the resources in this appendix to deepen your knowledge and supplement what you have read. Some of these sources have been mentioned in the preceding chapters. Many of these are additional sources of more specific or detailed information.

The New and Changing World of Work

- *We Are All Self Employed: The New Social Contract for Working in a Changing World.* Cliff Hakim, Berrett-Koehler Publishers, 1994. An excellent guide to shifting from an employee mentality to a self-employed attitude that includes methods of exploring what you want to do, what skills you bring to the marketplace, and who will be most interested in what you have to offer. This book will support and contribute to your growing awareness that there is no such thing as lifetime employment (job security), but there is lifetime employability (career security).

- *To Build the Life You Want, Create the Work You Love: the Spiritual Dimension of Entrepreneuring.* Marsha Sinetar, St. Martin's Press, 1995. The sequel to the best-selling and widely read book, *Do What You Love, The Money Will Follow.* This book will help you create work and/or understand the work you do from an inner-development standpoint in which "your consciousness is the doorway to the answers you want." Whether you are or intend to be an entrepreneur or want to apply their success strategies to your self-employed attitude as you work for others, you will find inspiration and explanation in this book. Topics include the seven qualities of ordinary people who take control of their working lives, the prerequisite mindset and attitude for success in uncharted and uncertain times, and how to replace job security with self-reliance.

- *C and the Box: A Paradigm Parable*. Frank A. Prince, Pfeiffer & Company, 1993. An illustrated story that helps you understand how the conditioning of your past can limit the potential of your future. In an entertaining and creative way, Prince demonstrates the importance of what happens when you get too comfortable with what is familiar and what it takes to explore new options in your professional and personal life.

- "The New Deal: What Companies and Employees Owe One Another." Brian O' Reilly, *Fortune* magazine, June 13, 1997. The cover story of this respected business publication explains why loyalty and job security are "nearly dead" and how employers who "deliver honesty and satisfying work can expect a new form of commitment form workers." This is an excellent overview of what has changed in employer-employee relationships in all industries, including healthcare.

- *Taking Responsibility: Self-Reliance and the Accountable Life*. Nathaniel Branden, Simon & Schuster, 1996. An important book for those wishing to broaden and deepen their knowledge of the concept of self-reliance and self-responsibility as it relates to strengthening the self for working and living differently as the 21st century dawns. Written by the psychologist who wrote the classic and best-selling book, *The Psychology of Self-Esteem*. Presents the critical importance of self-responsibility, self-reliance, and personal autonomy to the development of a healthy self in a newly emerging society in which personal strength and interdependence must coexist.

- *Job Shift: How to Prosper in a Workplace Without Jobs*. William Bridges, Addison-Wesley Publishing Company, 1994. This book is the source of a *Fortune* magazine cover story, "The End of the Job," and describes how organizations are transforming their employment structure from jobs, which represent artificial and overlapping divisions of responsibility, to work that needs to be done. Bridges encourages employees to respond to this shift by converting themselves into a business within a market, rather than remain on the payroll of one organization. A clear and concise guide to the facts as well as the psychological impact of "dejobbing," with specific information about how to run the business you have become which he calls "You & Co."

- "You, Inc.", *U.S. News & World Report*, October 28, 1996. A description of how America has "leapt headlong into the information age, and how careers will never be the same." The historical transition about the way in which work is organized and carried out is outlined, along with career profiles of people who have successfully made the transition to self-managing their careers by becoming "You, Inc., the fastest-growing employment segment in the economy." Chock full of useful data and tips, this article also has a section called "Twenty Hot Job Tracks," which includes healthcare and nursing opportunities.

- *Going Indie: Self Employment, Freelance, and Temping Opportunities.* Kathi Elster and Katherine Crowley, Simon & Schuster, 1997. Describes how "indies" (independently minded individuals) can take sole responsibility for generating their income and directing their careers, whether they consider themselves a temp, a part time worker, a freelance consultant, or a business owner. The ideas, tips, and trends in this book will help you shift from a paycheck mentality in which you rely on weekly paychecks and full-time benefits to a payroll mentality in which you pay yourself.

- *The Lifetime Career Manager: New Strategies for a New Era.* James C. Cabrera and Charles F. Albrecht, Jr, Adams Publishing Company, 1995. A comprehensive review of career planning information with an up-to-date look at how to manage your own career during the reengineering of corporate America. Challenges the myth of cradle-to-grave employment as it provides tips, guidelines, and ideas for shifting to the new employment reality of self-responsibility.

- *Liberation Management: Necessary Disorganization for the Nanosecond Nineties.* Tom Peters, Alfred A. Knopf, 1992. An outstanding and broad-reaching discussion of how the corporate and business world is "breaking themselves into bits" and reshaping everything about what they do and how they do it. Topics include why mergers are happening, the rise of "contract employment," and how careers are fast becoming "portfolios of jobs, on and off small or large firms' payrolls." Describes how the newly emerging and unsettling world of work and life in general "promises lots more room for growth, exercise of imagination, responsibility, and accountability than we have ever known before."

- *A Manager's Guide to the Millennium: Today's Strategies for Tomorrow's Success.* Ken Matejka and Richard J. Dunsing, American Management Association, 1995. An outstanding translation of how tomorrow's organizations will look and how to learn the new ground rules to "handle, enjoy, and even shape what's in store for you." Lives up to its description as a "millennium readiness manual" and is packed with action-oriented exercises to help you apply the strategies presented.

- *Healing the Wounds: Overcoming the Trauma of Layoffs and Revitalizing the Downsized Organizations.* David M. Noer, Jossey-Bass Publications, 1993. An indispensable guide to understanding the psychological and interpersonal impact of layoffs on work satisfaction and organizational productivity. Useful to staff and management levels of employees, this book includes such topics as how organizations are changing, the end of job security, the codependency problem, the layoff survivor (what happens to those who are left behind after downsizing), and how to empower people and build a new employment relationship.

General Career Guides

- *What Color is Your Parachute? A Practical Manual for Job-Hunters and Career Changers.* Richard Nelson Bolles, Ten Speed Press, 1998. Considered by many to be the classic guide and "bible" of career management across all industries, this book is updated annually with a new edition appearing each November. The 1998 guide is the 27th edition of this popular and eminently useful resource. Use this book to identify and utilize your skills more effectively whether you are job hunting or want to be more marketable in your current place of employment. You will find inspirational support as well as practical strategies related to interviewing, job hunting, and résumé writing.

- *Résumés! Résumés! Résumés!*, Second edition, Career Press, 1996. Top career experts from a variety of fields discuss and demonstrate how to compose effective résumés. Has an especially informative chapter relevant to the theme of this book called, "The Product? You. The Advertisement? Your Résumé." In addition to excellent information about the art of writing and editing a résumé, this book provides many samples from which to style your résumé.

- *Cover Letters! Cover Letters! Cover Letters!* Richard Fein, Career Press, 1994. This is an excellent guide to all business correspondence related to workplace and employment information, including cover letters, follow-up letters, and resignation letters. Also includes important information about networking, interviewing, and finding job leads.

- *I Could Do Anything if I Only Knew What It Was: How to Discover What You Really Want and How to Get It.* Barbara Sher, Dell Books, 1994. A guide and sourcebook for overcoming the blocks that prevent you from engaging in the work you want to be doing. This book takes you through a process of self-exploration, including action-oriented goal setting. Topics include "how to get off the fast track and on to the right track, first aid techniques for paralyzing chronic negativity, and how to regroup when you've lost your big dream."

- *Finding a Path With Heart: How to Go from Burnout to Bliss.* Beverly Potter, Ronin Publishers, 1995. A practical sourcebook that describes how to find work satisfaction, packed with entertaining and useful drawings, stories, exercises, and quotes. Helps in building self-reliance and includes topics like finding your path, defining your purpose, developing your vision, setting your goals, and transforming obstacles in your way.

- *The Third Wave: The Classic Study of Tomorrow.* Alvin Toffler, Bantam Books, 1980. Written by the futurist who wrote the often quoted classic, *Future Shock,* this book will help you understand how what we are currently experiencing as the Age of Information (the Third Wave) will forever change every area of our society. Toffler describes why the changes occurring today are different than anything that has happened in the recent past, and how this is only the third time in the entire history of mankind and civilization that a kind of change of this magnitude has occurred.

Managing Stress and Change In the New World of Work

- *Beat the Odds: Career Buoyancy Tactics for Today's Turbulent Job Market.* Martin Yate, Ballantine Books, 1995. A very readable and useful exploration of how to succeed in the changing world of work. Describes what is changing and why and provides practical suggestions for you to use. Topics include why layoffs aren't going to stop and what to do about it, the hot job opportunities, including healthcare, and developing such portable, core career competencies as goal orientation, positive expectancy, inner openness, personal influence, organized action, and informed risk.

- *Managing at the Speed of Change: How Resilient Managers Succeed and Prosper Where Others Fail.* Daryl R. Conner, Villard Books, 1994. Provides a structure and a practical approach to change while dealing with the feelings and behaviors common to the change experience. In addition to explaining what is changing and why in the world of work, this book will assist you in understanding the nature and process of change and translate these into specific strategies for coping effectively with stress.

- *Changing for Good: The Revolutionary Program That Explains the Six Stages of Change and Teaches You How to Free Yourself from Bad Habits,* James Prochaska, John Norcross, Carlo DiClemente, William Morrow and Co., 1994. A well organized approach to change with some refreshing reinterpretations that demystify the process and provide clear strategies for effective coping. Includes profiles of people coping effectively in each of the six stages of change as well as a helpful section on dealing with resistance to change itself.

- *Minding the Body, Mending the Mind,* Joan Borysenko, Bantam Books, Addison-Wesley Publishers, 1988. Written by a psychotherapist and scientist who is described as a pioneer in the new field of psychoneuroimmunology and the founder of the Mind Body Clinic at the New England Deaconess Hospital. This book provides sound and useful information on managing stress, as it explains the important relationship between mind and body.

- *Holistic Nursing: A Handbook for Practice,* Second Edition. Barbara Montgomery Dossey and Lynn Keegan, Aspen Publications, 1995. This is a stress management book disguised as a nursing textbook. Its approaches are useful for not only coping with stress in general, but with the particular kind of stress inherent in nursing practice. While it is the classic reference for the theory and practice of holistic nursing, its content is extremely relevant to every nurse who wants to understand and strengthen the healer aspect inherent in the nursing role and within the psyche of each nurse. It takes the reader on a inward journey towards wellness through self-discovery and personal reflection to achieve the goal of body, mind, and spirit wholeness. Packed with information about wellness, the psychophysiology of bodymind healing, nutrition, relaxation strategies, imagery, the authors assist you in consulting the truth within, and from that vantage point reach out more effectively to patients.

- *Resilience: How to Bounce Back When the Going Gets Tough,* Frederic Flach, Hatherleigh Press, 1997. A simple stress management guide with easy-to-understand descriptions of how stress happens and how to handle it. Topics include the response to stress at different points in the life cycle, what the resilient personality looks like, and how self-worth is related to resilience.

- *Kicking Your Stress Habits: A Do-It-Yourself Guide for Coping with Stress.* Donald A. Tubesing, Whole Person Associates, 1991. A simple and eminently useful self-study guide to stress and change management, with chapters devoted to perception, beliefs, grief, relationship skills, coping habits, and other topics.

- *Seeking Your Healthy Balance: A Do-It-Yourself Guide to Whole Person Well-Being.* Donald A. Tubesing, Whole Person Associates, 1991. Presents a holistic approach to taking care of yourself in the face of demands and responsibilities of work and family. Billed as a "workshop in a book," this resource provides such topics as how to juggle self and others, physical self-care, mental self-care, relational self-care, and spiritual self-care.

- *Thriving in Transition: Effective Living in Times of Change.* Marcia Perkins-Reed, Touchstone Books, Simon & Schuster, 1996. An easy-to-read and extremely useful book that explains how fundamental life changes will become an increasingly prevalent part of our lives, requiring a new attitude about the change experience as well as new skills to adapt to them. The author takes a holistic approach to the topic of change, using information from the fields of psychology, organizational development, physics, and spirituality. She uses this information to develop her own six-phase model of the transition process, including how to turn it into a time of growth.

- *Margin: Restoring Emotional, Physical, Financial, and Time Reserves to Overloaded Lives.* Richard A. Swenson, NavPress, 1992. This book can help you develop strategies for having too much to do and too little time to do it. Anxiety, stress, and eventual burnout can occur as change forces the closure of the space (margin) between ourselves and our limits, our reasonable workload and overload. This book combines the two important issues of time management and assertiveness in a creative new approach that will lead you to a new understanding of managing the responsibilities in your life.

Other Resources

- Various handbooks on managing organizational and personal change in the new world of work. Pritchett and Associates, Inc., 1997. Price Pritchett and his consultancy group publish handbooks based on their training seminars, which cover a wide variety of issues relevant to understanding organizational change and its impact on productivity, interpersonal relationships, and personal stress. These low-cost handbooks translate complicated concepts into understandable and useful strategies and are applicable to management and staff levels of personnel. Handbook titles include:

  Firing Up Commitment During Organizational Change

  The Stress of Organizational Change

  Team Reconstruction: Building a High Performance Work Group During Change

  The Employee Handbook for Organizational Change

  Culture Shift: Survival of the Fittest, New Work Habits for a Radically Changing World

  High Velocity Culture Change: A Handbook for Managers

    Contact: Pritchett and Associates, Inc., 13155 Noel Road, Suite 1600, Dallas, TX 75240; (214) 789-7900.

- Self-study handbooks published by Crisp Publications for learning about business and personal issues relevant to living and working effectively. Subject areas include management, human resources, communication skills, personal development, organizational development, and stress management. The books average 70 to 90 pages in length, are written by authorities in their fields, and are packed with exercises and self-assessment tools to help you cope more effectively with change. Titles include:

Managing Personal Change: A Primer for Today's World by Cynthia D. Scott and Dennis Jaffe

Managing Organizational Change: A Practical Guide for Managers by Cynthia D. Scott and Dennis Jaffe

Understanding Organizational Change: Converting Theory to Practice by Lynn Fossum

Managing Disagreement Constructively: Conflict Management in Organizations by Herbert S. Kindler

Personal Time Management by Marion E. Haynes

Managing Anger: Methods for a Happier and Healthier Life by Rebessa R. Luhn

Finding Your Purpose: A Guide to Personal Fulfillment by Barbara J. Braham

Developing Self Esteem: A Guide for Positive Success by Connie Palladino

Developing Positive Assertiveness: Practical Techniques for Personal Success by Sam R., Lloyd

Self-Empowerment: Getting What You Want From Life by Sam R. Lloyd and Tina Berthelot

Empowerment: A Practical Guide For Success By Cynthia D. Scott, Ph.D., M.P.H., and Dennis T. Jaffe, Ph.D.

Effective Networking: Proven Techniques for Career Success by Venda Rahy-Johnson

Contact: Crisp Publications, Inc., 1200 Hamilton Court, Menlo Park, CA 94025; (800) 442-7477.

Personal Growth, Development, and Self-Awareness

- *The 7 Habits of Highly Effective People: Powerful Lessons in Personal Change.* Stephen R. Covey, Simon & Schuster, 1990. A well known and widely read classic that presents a "principal-centered" approach for solving professional and personal issues. This approach can lead you to developing the inner security you need for adapting to change as well as "taking advantage of the opportunities that change creates."

- *Principle-Centered Leadership.* Stephen R. Covey, Summit Books, 1991. Explores issues of personal development that lead to spending your time around self-identified principles rather than the priorities of others. Personal fulfillment and professional success emerge as a result of answering questions such as how to achieve balance between work and family, how to unleash creative talent, and how to develop and use your mission statement.

- *First Things First.* Stephen R. Covey, A. Roger Merrill, and Rebecca R. Merrill, Simon & Schuster, 1994. A time-management book that expands on and specifies Covey's time-management description in *The 7 Habits of Highly Effective People.* Correlates time management with vision, roles, and empowerment principles. In doing so, the book goes way beyond the usual lists for learning to manage yourself.

- *Developing a 21st Century Mind.* Marsha Sinetar, Villard Books, 1991. This best-selling author of *Do What You Love, the Money Will Follow* describes a process she calls positive structuring, the necessary path to shifting from the traditional mind—which Sinetar argues is fear-motivated, dualistic, and ego-centric—to the nondualistic and synergistic 21st century mind needed for living successfully as the world changes and demands new attitudes and behaviors from everyone. An excellent guide to understanding and facilitating personal development as well as interdependence.

- *Emotional Intelligence: Why it Can Matter More Than IQ.* Daniel Goleman, Bantam Books, 1995. No exploration of personal growth and development is complete without an understanding of emotions and feelings and their impact on self and others. This book, fast becoming a classic in its field, presents ground-breaking behavioral research that explains and demonstrates how emotional intelligence is essential to self awareness, impulse control, self-discipline, persistence, self-motivation, and empathy.

- *The Fifth Discipline Fieldbook: Strategies and Tools for Building a Learning Organization.* Peter Senge, Currency and Doubleday Books, 1994. A beautifully conceived and organized book based on Senge's classic work, *The Fifth Discipline*, which introduced the concept of how organizations and the individuals in them need to learn in order to be effective, especially as the world of work changes. Topics include reinventing relationships, building vision, developing personal mastery, and systems thinking. Packed with useful exercises for self-exploration and the building of skills.

- *The Path of Least Resistance: Learning to Become the Creative Force in Your Own Life.* Robert Fritz, Fawcett Columbine Publishers, 1989. Explains how to move into your future vision by understanding your present reality and using the creative tension between these two experiences to create the momentum you need to get where you want to go.

- *Women Who Run With the Wolves: Myths and Stories of the Wild Woman Archetype.* Clarissa Pinkola Estes, Ballantine Books, 1992. This book invites you to experience the powerful force within you that is "natural, creative, powerful, filled with good instincts and ageless knowing." Written by a Jungian analyst and storyteller, you will participate in "psychic archeological digs" into the female unconscious by way of stories like "Bluebeard" and "The Little Match Girl." Nurses will especially identify with the chapter called "Homing: Returning to OneSelf."

- *Revolution from Within: A Book of Self-Esteem.* Gloria Steinem, Little, Brown, and Co., 1992. An autobiographical account of this feminist's life and journey, primarily from the standpoint of her own personal development. She suggests that the social revolution in which she has been engaged most of her life is only one half of what is needed for change to come about. The other revolution needs to come from within each person, a necessary "revolution of spirit and consciousness" which she had always assumed was either secondary or inconsequential to social change.

- *Pro-Nurse Handbook: Designed for the Nurse Who Wants to Survive/Thrive Professionally.* Melodie Chenevert, Mosby, 1993. An entertaining and useful guide to understanding and managing the personal and interpersonal problems that lead to the loss of work satisfaction and sometimes to burnout. Packed with scenarios familiar to every nurse along with tips and strategies needed to think and act differently. Topics include learning to pace yourself, ways to increase your work satisfaction, dealing with procrastination, and understanding the "business" of nursing.

- *Healing Yourself: A Nurse's Guide to Self-Care and Renewal.* Sherry Kahn and Mileva Saulo, Delmar Publishers, Inc., 1994. A concise and comprehensive handbook with holistic approaches that are practical and easy to use in order to sustain your "body, mind, and spirit as you meet the daily demands of your challenging career." Covers such stress reduction techniques as breathing, exercise, nutrition, and self massage, as well as emotions and their role in stress, the causes and effects of stress, and relevant body-mind research.

- *A Passion For the Possible: A Guide to Realizing Your True Potential.* Jean Houston, Harper San Francisco, 1997. Creates an understanding of how to break free from the limiting beliefs that will prevent you from taking advantage of the opportunities change always brings. Considered by many to be a great teacher and writer, Houston uses her vast psychological, spiritual, and mythic knowledge to lead you on a journey of self-discovery that will leave you feeling more optimistic about your potential and the possibilities that can await you in the changing world.

- *Self Renewal: High Performance in a High Stress World.* Dennis T. Jaffe and Cynthia D. Scott, Crisp Publications, 1994. An extremely useful workbook that contains clear explanations as well as self-assessment tools and self-reflection exercises. Uses a self care approach to stress management, presenting ways to increase your self-awareness, self-management, and self-renewal strategies.

- *Jesus, CEO: Using Ancient Wisdom for Visionary Leadership*. Laurie Beth Jones, Hyperion Books, 1995. Written by the author of *The Path*, this deceptively simple book presents a powerful and extremely useful approach to empowering yourself no matter what your level of leadership, whether you are a leader of others or just a leader of yourself. Jones presents strategies for attaining the three strengths present in the leadership of Jesus—self-mastery, action, and relationships—and uses the life of Jesus as a model to be emulated. She describes how "Jesus, a "CEO" took a disorganized "staff" of twelve and built "a thriving enterprise." This is a fresh and humor-filled approach to motivating and empowering yourself.

- *The Artist's Way: A Spiritual Path to Higher Creativity*. Julia Cameron, G. P. Putnam Sons, 1992. An empowering book to increase the creative expression of any and all areas of your life. Engages you in a 12-week personal development journey to "recover your creativity from a variety of blocks, including limiting beliefs, fear, self sabotage, jealousy, guilt, addictions, and other inhibiting forces." Based on the popular and highly effective 12-week course by the same name offered in various parts of the country.

- *The Path: Creating Your Mission Statement for Work and for Life*. Laurie Beth Jones, Hyperion, 1996. Provides inspiring and practical advice to lead readers through the steps of defining and fulfilling a mission in life. The lessons on creating a mission statement are easily transferable to the world of work.

- *Life Skills: Taking Charge of Your Personal and Professional Growth*. Richard J. Leider, Pfeiffer & Company, 1994. Takes a personal development viewpoint to career strategies and work success. Life and work planning are explored in an interactive workbook to "help you align your career objectives, talents, and deepest values." Topics include organizing your life and work priorities, establishing a governing purpose and values, and understanding your personal life vision.

- *Use Your Anger: A Woman's Guide to Empowerment.* Sandra Thomas and Cheryl Jefferson, Pocket Books, Simon and Schuster, 1996. Written by a nurse and based on a seven-year, nationwide study she conducted, this book will help you understand the impact anger may be having on your life and provides your with ways to transform the energy of anger into productive and empowering action. Through questionnaires and special exercises, you can explore your anger triggers, anger style, anger tactics, anger reactions, and anger strategies.

Trends, Predictions, and Statistics

- *Power Shift: Knowledge, Wealth, and Violence as the Edge of the 21st Century.* Alvin Toffler, Bantam Books, 1990. Written by a world-famous and widely respected futurist and scholar, this book provides an extensive exploration of the tremendous shifts in power taking place globally and locally. These shifts are affecting everything we do, see, and are influenced by, including the world of supermarkets, hospitals, banks, businesses, offices, and television. Describes what is changing in our culture, why it's changing, and how to rethink choices in a world based on information and knowledge.

- *Megatrends: Ten New Directions Transforming Our Lives.* John Naisbitt, Warner Books, 1986. The classic and oft-quoted book about the period of great changes and transisiton that the United States is presently experiencing as it shifts from industrial production to providing service and information. An excellent resource to help you understand how and why we are moving from an industrial to an information society, from institutional help to self-help, and from hierarchies to networking.

- *Megatrends for Women.* Patricia Aburdene and John Naisbitt, Villard Books, 1992. These international social forecasters describe how "the women of the 1990s are challenging the male-dominated status quo, reintegrating female values and perspectives and recasting the social, political, and economic megatrends of the day." The social, political, and economic influences that continue to support this trend are discussed. This issue has an obvious and inescapable impact on the values and practice of the female-dominated profession of nursing.

- *The Popcorn Report: Faith Popcorn on the Future of Your Company, Your World, Your Life.* Faith Popcorn, Doubleday, 1992. An indispensable and simply written guide with a bit of lightness thrown in for understanding the mind-numbing changes seizing the world at the beginning of the 21st century. Faith Popcorn, called the "Nostradamus of Marketing" by *Fortune* magazine, explains what the future will look like and how to profit from it. She explains "what we will buy, where we will work, and what we will think in the next decade."

- *Clicking: Sixteen Trends to Future-Fit Your Life, Your Work, and Your Business.* Faith Popcorn and Lys Marigold, Harper Collins, 1996. By the futurist and author of the often-quoted *Popcorn Report*, this book continues the authors ideas and predictions about the business and persoanl trends that are and will be shaping every aspect of our lives. Here you will find the strategies you need to fit yourself into the new careers and lifestyles of today and the future.

- *Workplace 2000: The Revolution Reshaping American Business.* Joseph Boyett and Henry P. Conn, Plume Books, 1991. An excellent description of what the future American workplace will look like and what employees need to do to meet the new demands and expectations. Topics include how middle management will be replaced with self-directed work teams, the difference between managers and leaders, and how and why employees must learn self management.

- *Occupational Outlook Handbook.* United States Department of Labor, Bureau of Labor Statistics, U.S. Government Printing Office, 1996. An essential guide to how all occupations are affected by the dramatic and sweeping changes of the late 1990s, including a listing and description of growth industries such as healthcare.

Nursing-Specific Career Guidance

- "Creating Your Mission Statement for Work and for Life." Paula Schneider, *Nursing Spectrum*, Gannett Satellite Information Network, Inc., 1998. Written by a registered nurse who studied with Laurie Beth Jones, author of *The Path*: *Creating Your Mission Statement for Work and For Life*. This article summarizes the process of creating your mission statement and includes examples of its application to nursing.

- *What You Need to Know About Today's Workplace: A Survival Guide for Nurses* Lyndia Flanagan, American Nurses Publishing, 1995. In addition to explaining how and why the healthcare industry is changing, this book provides useful information about employment rights and protections (such as collective bargaining, at-will employment, and layoffs), employer terms and conditions of employment (such as performance appraisals, grievance handling, and liability protection), and the management of stress and conflicts in restructuring environments. There is an extensive appendix with sources of information on employment rights and protections as well as a comprehensive reference list and bibliography. Flanagan encourages nurses to become "sophisticated about survival and growth in an industry playing under new ground rules by becoming business-minded professionals, more effective leaders in the workplace, and more discerning employees."

- "Career Alternatives For Nurses." Donna Cardillo, Cardillo & Associates, 1996. This video is based on the workshop of the same name conducted by the author. It presents and reviews nursing roles most relevant to the changing healthcare marketplace and describes the settings in which they are most likely to be found.

- *Career Guidance for Nurses*. Clarissa Russo, Russo & Associates, 1990. This workbook and accompanying audio cassette is based on a popular and very informative nursing career seminar given by a nurse who specializes in nursing career alternatives and self-marketing strategies. Contains many useful self-reflection exercises to guide you through the process of taking charge of and directing your nursing career. Topics include sorting out career satisfactions and dissatisfactions, converting fears into action and success, and career alternatives to consider.

• *Marketing Ourselves: Things We Never Learned in Nursing School.* Clarissa Russo, Russo & Associates, 1990. Topics of interest include the power of imagining your possibilites, how to set and attain goals, and tips on getting started in your own business. Also included are many articles written by the author that appeared elsewhere.

• *Nursing Spectrum 1997 Career Fitness Guide.* Gannett Satellite Information Network, Inc. This is an excellent resource by the publishers of Nursing Spectrum magazine. The many nationwide advertisements provide you with excellent information about the features, professional climate, and changing purpose and structure of the organizations. This book will prove very useful as healthcare continues to restructure, and contains important addresses and phone numbers. In addition, there are many useful career-oriented articles on such topics as how to discover new sources of satisfaction at work, how to survive conflict, how to network, and what career success will look like in the next millennium. A resources section is also included, providing lists of nursing specialty organizations, certification resources, and state boards of nursing.

• *Tomorrow's Solution for Today's Nurse: The Nursing Career Development Process.* New York State Nurses Association, 1997. A workbook of career development information that summarizes the issues facing nurses as a result of the present and predicted changes in healthcare. Based on applying the cornerstone components of the nursing process with which you are familiar, this handbook will guide you through the similar series of logical steps so that you can assess your needs and develop an effective career and employment plan. Contains an excellent list of career resources, including general and nursing-specific information.

• *The Pfizer Guide: Nursing Career Opportunities.* Published for the Pfizer Laboratories, Pratt, and Roerig divisions of Pfizer, Inc., by Merritt Communications, 1994. Edited by Mary O. Mundinger. A compendium of over 50 nursing career profiles written by nurses who specialize in each of the roles they write about. Contains detailed information about the role, practice environments, and qualifications necessary to pursue each as a career path. An excellent guide for nurses seeking to understand the almost endless variations of nursing experiences and specialties whether seeking a new role in nursing or wanting to strengthen the role you already have.

- *Reinventing Your Nursing Career: A Handbook for Success in the Age of Managed Care.* Michael Newell and Mario Pinardo, Aspen Publications, 1998. Describes how and why nursing and healthcare is changing with special emphasis on the managed care opportunities and the healthcare industry as a consumer-driven business environment. Additional features include a discussion of the process of personal empowerment and strategies for coping with change.

- *Managing Your Career in Nursing.* Frances C. Henderson and Barbara O. McGettigan, National League for Nursing Press, 1994. Provides specific and very detailed descriptions about traditional and emerging nursing practice options and opportunities, including self-assessment tools for practically every topic discussed. Nursing novices as well as seasoned professionals who seek a detailed understanding of nursing roles will find this book helpful. Also contains excellent resource sections and well-documented trends and predictions about the changing healthcare industry.

Understanding the Changing Healthcare Industry

- *Nurse Case Management in the 21st Century.* Edited by Elaine L. Cohen, Mosby Publishing Company, 1996. An outstanding group of essays packed full of information about the changing healthcare system with contributions from some of the most knowledgeable and influential nurse leaders and futurists, including Tim Porter-O'Grady. An indispensable guide for those plotting a career path in case management as well as nurses who want to enhance their knowledge about the emerging role of the nurse along the Continuum of Care.

- *Life After Downsizing: Strategies for Organizational Healing and Revitalization.* Rosalle A. Tyrrell, MedSurg Nursing, 1994. Provides structured interventions necessary for restoring the personal and interpersonal health and well-being of the organization in this age of downsizing.

- "Layoff Survivor Sickness: Minimizing the Sequelae of Organizational Transformation." Pamela Klauer Triolo, *Journal of the Organization of Nurse Administrators*, March 1996. An excellent article that applies David Noer's seminal work on layoff survivor sickness to nursing and healthcare settings. In addition to summarizing pertinent information from Noer's book, *Healing The Wounds: Overcoming the Trauma of Layoffs and Revitalizing the Downsized Organizations*, the author provides specific strategies helpful to nurses practicing at any level.

- *Reengineering Nursing and Healthcare: The Handbook for Organizational Transformation.* Suzanne Smith Blancett and Dominick L. Flarey, Aspen Publishers, 1995. This text adapts the framework of the bestselling book, Reengineering the Corporation and applies its principles to understanding how and why healthcare is changing from compartmentalized services to more seamlessly integrated systems. Essential for nurse managers and leadership nurses in general, and to all nurses who want an in-depth understanding of the process of hospital and healthcare reengineering.

- *Who's Who in Health: A Guide to New York Area Companies and Service Providers.* Crain's New York Business, Crain Communication, Inc., 1998. Provides an annual, up-to-date guide to and information about the New York healthcare community, including hospitals, insurers, consumer information, physician groups, and business services. An important resource for those living in or considering relocating to the New York area, as well as an excellent example of a regional publication that is duplicated in other forms through out the country.

Computer And Internet Resources

- American Nurses Association, Council for Nursing Services and Informatics, 600 Maryland Avenue SW, Washington DC 20024-2571; (202) 651-7000

- Midwest Alliance for Nursing Informatics, P.O. Box 9313, Downers Grove, IL 60515; 708-923-4535

- *Nurses Guide to the Internet.* Leslie H. Nicoll and Teena H. Ouellette, Lippincott, 1997. A handbook with information about using the Internet, specifically targeted to nurses. Packed with useful information about the Internet in general, how to get started, how to access Listserv groups, use e-mail for networking, conduct research, and use bulletin boards. Internet addresses are included in the book's directory of sites along with a description of each and its usefulness to you.

- *Computers in Nursing.* Edited by Leslie H. Nicoll, Lippincott Publishers. A bimonthly journal of practical information about effect of and application of computer technology in nursing practice and in general healthcare.

- American Medical Informatics Association—Nursing Informatics Working Group. Promotes the advancement of nursing informatics within the larger multidisciplinary context of health informatics. Publishes a semiannual electronic newsletter designed to keep the nursing community up to date with the changing healthcare informatics environment. To subscribe, send an e-mail message to abbott@gl.umbc.edu.

- *Informatics Nurse Certification Catalogue.* American Nurses Credentialing Center, Washington, D.C.

- *Nursing Informatics: Where Caring and Technology Meet.* M. J. Ball, K. J. Hannah, S. K. Newbold, and J. K. Douglas, Second Edition, Springer-Verlag, 1995.

- *Introduction to Nursing Informatics.* K.J. Hannah, M.J. Ball, and M. Edwards, Springer-Verlag, 1994.

Internet Web Sites

Information Specific to Nursing

- *NetNurse* (http://www.wp.com/NetNurse/home.html). Links nurses to the World Wide Web, including nurses' home pages, schools of nursing, support groups, and search engines.

- *NP Web* (http://www.unh.edu/). Provides resources to assist nurse practitioners in accessing medical and healthcare sites as well as links to networking and career related information.

- *Nurse WWW Information Server* (http://medsrv2.bham.ac.uk/nursing/). Provides links to a wide variety of nursing Internet resources, including the electronic journal, *Nursing Standard Online.*

- *Nurses' Call* (http://www.npl.com/~nrs_call/). Provides conference and convention announcements, employment listings, and information about prominent nurses on the Internet.

- *Nurseweek* (http://www-nurseweek.webnexus.com). Provides a forum for nurses to exchange ideas and information related to local, regional, and national issues, healthcare news, resources, and employment opportunities.

- *NurseWIRE* (http://www.callamer.com/itc/nursewire/). Provides lists of nurse entrepreneurs using the Internet in enterprising ways to promote and inform others of their business.

- *Nursing* (http://www.lib.umich.edu/tml/nursing/html). Provides information about and links to career information, clinical nursing resources, discussion forums, professional associations, and electronic journals.

- *Nursing NCLEX* (http://www.kaplan.com:80/nclex/). The Internet site of Kaplan Educational Centers, which provides NCLEX review courses as well as information related to nursing careers and job opportunities. Also provides links to educational and testing materials for the GMAT, MCAT, and GRE for nurses considering graduate education.

- *Nursing Network Forum* (http://www.access.digex.net/~nurse/nursnet#.htm). The nursing Internet site of the Microsoft Network, which provides comprehensive and worldwide networking and information about all aspects of nursing practice. This is a high-volume site that is interesting and extremely easy to use.

- *NursingNet* (http://www.communique.net/~nursgnt/). Provides networking forum for students, nursing, and medical professionals to disseminate information to each other and to the public about health-related topics.

- *SpringNet* (http://www.springnet.com). Maintained by the Springhouse Corporation, publishers of the well-known journals and books: Nursing '98, Nursing Manangement, The Nurse Practitioner, and Nursing '99 Drug Handbook. In addition to information about and from these publications, they provide a reference library, employment opportunities, online networking events, continuing education, and conference listings.

- *Nursing Center* (http://www.nursingcenter.com). Maintained by Lippincott Publishers, a well-known publishing house for nursing books and journals, including the American Journal of Nursing. Provides networking, career, and clinical information, including a career center, online networking, and continuing education.

- *Nursing Spectrum* Career Fitness (http://www.nursingspectrum.com). The online resource to this well known and eminently useful employment and career-oriented publication. Provides chat rooms, a bookstore, employment listings, including instant applications and résumé submission, self-study modules for continuing education credit, employer profiles, and a weekly online guest lecture.

General Career Assistance

- *Career Mosaic* (http://www.careermosaic.com/cm). A wide variety of career support)

- *CareerPath* (http://www.careerpath.com/res/owa/rb_applicant.display_rblogin?). A national employment site containing lists from the nation's leading newspapers and employers, cited to have the largest volume and most current job listings.

- *America's Job Bank* (http://www.ajb.dni.us/). An employment site with a wide variety of national job listings, including job market information, employer information, and search tips.

- *The Job Network* (http://www.conquest-prod.com/resume.html). Provides free searches, job postings, and resume postings).

- *The Catapult* (http://www.jobweb.org/catapult/catapult.html). A springboard to many job sites and resources.

- *Job Web* (http://www.jobweb.org). A wide variety of career support.

- *Nation Job Network* (http://www.nationjob.com). A wide variety of career support and networking advice.

- *Online Career Center* (http//www.occ.com). A wide variety of career support.

- *Top Secrets of Résumé Writing* (http//www.amsquare.com:80/america/amer-way/res21ndz.htm)

E-Mail Distribution Lists (Listservs)

- *NRSING-L* (listproc@lists.umass.edu). Provides a discussion list on nursing informatics.

- *NRSINGED* (listserv@ulkyvm.louisville.edu). Provides a discussion list on nursing education, probably of greatest use to nurse educators.

- *NURSENET* (listserv@listserv.utoronto.ca). Provides an international electronic forum for the discussion of a wide variety of nursing practice and clinical issues.

- *SNURSE* (listserv@ubvm.ccbuffalo.edu). Provides forums and discussion groups for student nurses.

Professional Nursing Associations and Organizations

Case Management

- Case Management Society of America, 1101 17th Street NW, Suite 1200, Washington, DC 20036; (202) 296-9200

- Association of Medical Case Managers, 6101 Ball Road, Suite 102, Cypress, CA 90630; (703) 220-0815

Advanced Nursing Practice

- American Academy of Nurse Practitioners, PO Box 12846, Austin, TX 78711; (512) 442-4262

- American Association of Nurse Anesthetists, 222 South Prospect Avenue, Park Ridge, IL 60068; (847) 692-7050

- American College of Nurse Midwives, 818 Connecticut Avenue, NW Suite 900, Washington, DC; (800) 753-2266

Entrepreneurial Nursing

- National Nurses in Business Association, Staten Island, NY (800) 331-6534

Home Health Care

- National Association for Home Care, 519 C Street NE, Washington, DC 20002; (202) 547-7424

Hospice Care

- The Hospice Association of America, 519 C Street NE, Washington, DC 20002; (202) 547-7424

- National Hospice Organization, 1901 North Moore Street, Arlington, VA 22209; (703) 243-5900

Holistic Nursing

- American Holistic Nurses Association, P.O. Box 2130, Flagstaff, AZ 86003; (520) 526-2196

- National Association of Nurse Massage Therapists, P.O. Box 1150, Abita Springs, LA 70420; (707) 762-5588

Medical-Surgical Nursing and Related Fields

- Academy of Medical Surgical Nurses, E. Holly Ave., Box 56, Pitman, NJ 08071; (609) 256-2323

- American Assoication of Diabetes Educators, 100 W. Monroe, Fourth Floor, Chicago, IL 60603; (312) 424-2426

- Oncology Nursing Society, 501 Holiday Drive, Pittsburgh, PA 15220; (850) 474-8869

- Wound, Ostomy, and Continence Nurses Society, 1550 S. Coast Highway, Suite 201, Laguna Beach, CA 92651; (888) 224-7262

- American Association of Spinal Cord Injury Nurses, 75-20 Astoria Blvd., Jackson Heights, NY 11370; (718) 803-3782

- American Society of Pain Management Nurses, 7794 Grow Drive, Pensacola, FL 32514; (850) 484-8762

- Association for Practitioners in Infection Control, 1016 16th St. NW, Sixth Floor, Washington, DC 20036; (202) 296-2742

- Association of Nurses in AIDS Care, 11250 Roger Bacon Dr., Suite B, Reston, VA 20190; (703) 925-0081

- Intravenous Nurses Association, 10 Fawcett St. Third Floor, Cambridge, MA 02138; (617) 331-3008

Perioperative Nursing

- Association of Operating Room Nurses, 3170 S. Parker Rd., Suite 300, Denver CO 80231; (303) 755-6300

Pediatric Nursing

- Association of Pediatric Oncology Nurses, 4700 West Lake Ave., Glenview, IL 60025; (847) 375-4724

Legal Nurse Consulting

- American Association of Legal Nurse Consultants, 4700 W. Lake Ave., Glenview, IL 60025; (847)375-4713

- Amerian Association of Nurse Attorneys, 3525 Ellicott Mills Dr. Suite N, Ellicott City, MD 21043; (410) 418-4800

Ambulatory Care Nursing

- American Academy of Ambulatory Care Nurses, E. Holly Ave., Box 56, Pitman, NJ 08071; (609) 256-2350

- American Association of Office Nurses, 109 Kinderkamack Rd., Montvale, NJ 07645; (201) 391-2600

Occupational Health Nursing

- American Assoicaiton of Occupational Health Nurses, Inc., 2920 Brandywine Rd., Suite 100, Atlanta, GA 30341; (770) 455-7757

School Nursing

- National Association of School Nurses, P.O. Box 1300, Scarborough, ME 04070; (207) 883-2117

Gerontological Nursing

- National Gerontological Nursing Association, 7250 Parkway Drive, Suite 510, E. Holly Ave. Box 56, Pitman, NJ 08071; (609) 256-2333

National and State Nursing Organizations and Associations

Note: National associations can supply contact information for state associations. For example, the American Nurses Association will provide information about each of its 50 state-affiliated associations.

- American Nurses Association, 600 Maryland Ave. SW, Suite 100 West, Washington, DC 20024; (202) 651-7000

- American Academy of Nursing, 600 Maryland Ave. SW, Suite 100 West, Washington, DC 20024; (202) 651-7238

- National League for Nursing, 350 Hudson Street, New York, NY 10014; (212) 989-9393

- The National Student Nurse Association, 555 West 57th Street, Suite 1327, New York, NY 10019; (212) 581-2368

Psychiatric Mental-Health Nursing and Related Fields

- Drug and Alcohol Nursing Association, Inc., 660 Lonely Cottage Dr., Upper Black Eddy, PA 18972; (610) 847-5396

- National Nurses Society on Addictions, 4101 Lake Boone Trail, Suite 201, Raleigh, NC 27607; (919) 783-5871

- American Psychiatric Nurses Association, 1200 19th Street, NW, Suite 300, Washington, DC 20036; (202) 857-1133

Nursing Management and Administration

- American Organization of Nurse Executives, One North Franklin, 34th Floor, Chicago, IL 60606; (312) 422-2800

Rehabilitation and Long-Term Care Nursing

- American Society for Long-Term Care Nurses, 660 Lonely Cottage Dr., Upper Black Eddy, PA 18972; (610) 847-5063

- Association of Rehabilitation Nurses, 4700 W. Lake Ave., Glenview, IL 60025; (847) 375-4777

Men in Nursing

- American Assembly for Men in Nursing, c/o NYSNA, 11 Cornell Rd., Latham, NY 12110; (518) 782-9530

Nursing Education

- American Association of Colleges in Nursing, One Dupont Circle, NW, Suite 530, Washington, DC 20036; (202) 463-6930

- National Nursing Staff Development Organization, 7794 Grow Drive, Pensacola, FL 32514; (850) 474-8762

Critical Care Nursing and Related Fields

- Emergency Nurses Association, 216 Higgins Road, Park Ridge, IL 60068; (854) 698-9400

- American Association of Critical Care Nurses, 101 Columbia, Alisa Viejo, CA 92656; (714) 363-2020

Obstetrical and Womens Health Nursing

- Association of Women's Health, Obstetric, and Neonatal Nursing, 700 14th Street NW, Suite 600, Washington, DC 20005; (202) 737-0575

Certification

- American Nurses Credentialing Center, 600 Maryland Avenue S.W., Suite 100 West, Washington DC 20024; (800) 284-2378

In addition, contact nursing specialty organizations such as the American Association of Critical Care Nurses to determine if they grant board certification in their specialty.

Journals and Publications

Contact the nursing specialty association of interest to you to subscribe to their specific journals, publications, and newsletters. For example, The Association of Critical Care Nurses publishes an excellent and widely read journal called *Critical Care Nursing*.

- *The American Nurse.* This bimonthly newsletter, published by the American Nurses Association, is an important source of nursing practice news, including political/legislative issues, employment practices, workplace issues, and convention news. Members of the American Nurses Association and its 50 affiliated state associations receive this newsletter as a part of their membership.

- *Report.* This official newsletter of the New York State Nurses Association contains state-wide information about nursing practice issues, just as The American Nurse (described above) provides issues of national interest and concern. Each state nurses association publishes an official newsletter with a different title. Contact your state association for information. Membership in ANA and your state nurses association entitles you to a subscription.

- *Calendar.* This official newsletter of the New York Counties Registered Nurses Association, District 13 of the New York State Nurses Association contains district-wide information about nursing practice issues, just as The American

Nurse (described above) provides issues of national interest and concern, and Report provides state-wide issues. Each state nurses association is divided into a number of districts and each publishes an official newsletter with a different title. Contact your state association for information on these district publications. Membership in ANA and your state nurses association entitles you to a subscription.

- *The American Journal of Nursing* (AJN). Monthly journal published by Lippincott for The American Nurses Association (ANA), considered the official voice of the ANA, and therefore an important source of nursing practice information. In addition to news about nursing practice issues, AJN provides comprehensive and in-depth clinical articles, including the ability to earn continuing education units by answering and submitting test questions following some of its articles. Members of the American Nurses Association and its 50 affiliated state associations receive this journal as a part of their membership.

- *Nursing 98.* Published by the Springhouse Corporation. This is a leading source of practical clinical and professional information, continuing education, and current news about drugs, equipment, and techniques for nurses who are direct caregivers. The journal also offers insight into the human and professional sides of nursing.

- *Nursing Management.* Published by the Springhouse Corporation, this widely read journal is an indispensable guide to understanding nursing management and healthcare administration, whether you are a manager or just want to understand and keep abreast of current nursing/healthcare management issues.

- *Nursing Spectrum.* Published biweekly by Gannett Satellite Information Network, Nursing Spectrum is the New York metropolitan area's version of an employment and career-oriented publication that is circulated under different names in other areas of the country. This publication is available free to all licensed professional nurses. It contains employment opportunities and career/workplace information that will help you keep abreast of changes and issues in nursing practice and healthcare.

State Licensing Requirements

Alabama

Board of Nursing
RSA Plaza, Suite 250
770 Washington Avenue
Montgomery, AL 36130-3900
(334) 242-4060
Temporary Permit: 90 days from date of graduation; three months if by endorsement. $50
State Board Fee: $85 R.N., $75 L.P.N.
Additional State Endorsement: $80 R.N., $70 L.P.N.
NCLEX Test Fee: $88
Re-Examination Limitations: None
License Renewal: Every even year on December 31 for R.N.'s; Every odd year on December 31 for L.P.N.'s. $60
CEU Requirements: 24 hours per renewal period

Alaska

Board of Nursing
Dept. of Commerce
Div. of Occupational Licensing
P.O. Box 110806
Juneau, AK 99811-0806
(907) 465-2544
Temporary Permit: Four months if by endorsement. $50
State Board Fee: $155
Additional State Endorsement: $105
NCLEX Test Fee: $88
Re-Examination Limitations: Must pass within 5 years, then retake with remediation
License Renewal: Every even year on November 30 (R.N.). $105
CEU Requirements: Two of the three required for renewal: (1) 30 contact hours of CE, (2) 30 hours of

professional nursing activities, (3) 320 hours of nursing employment

Arizona

Board of Nursing
1651 E. Morten Avenue, Suite 150
Phoenix, AZ 85020
(602) 331-8111
Temporary Permit: Two months, no permit by exam. $25
State Board Fee: $135
Additional State Endorsement: $70
Re-Examination Limitations: Four times within one year
License Renewal: Birthday, every two years. $50
CEU Requirements: None

Arkansas

State Board of Nursing
Univ. Tower Bldg.
1123 S. Univ. Avenue, Suite 4030
Little Rock, AR 72204
(501) 686-2700
Temporary Permit: Up to 90 days if by endorsement and advanced practice, $10
State Board Fee: $55
Additional State Endorsement: $75
NCLEX Test Fee: $88
Re-Examination Limitations: None
License Renewal: Birthday, every two years. $25
CEU Requirements: None

California

Board of Registered Nursing
400 R Street, Suite 4030
Sacramento, CA 95814
(916) 322-3350
Temporary Permit: Interim license pending results of first exam; six months if by endorsement, $30
State Board Fee: $75 application fee, $32 fingerprint fee
Additional State Endorsement: $50, $56 fingerprint fee
NCLEX Test Fee: $88 ($97.25 by mail)
Re-Examination Limitations: None
License Renewal: Every two years, on the last day of the month following birth month. $80
CEU Requirements: All R.N.s: 30 contact hours every two years

Colorado

Board of Nursing
1560 Broadway, Suite 670
Denver, CO 80202
(303) 894-2430
Temporary Permit: 90 days; four months if by endorsement. Fee is included in application fee.
State Board Fee: $66
Additional State Endorsement: $76
NCLEX Test Fee: $88
Re-Examination Limitations: None

License Renewal: Every two years, $68
CEU Requirements: None

Connecticut

Department of Public Health
Nurse Licensure
410 Capitol Avenue, MS 12 APP
P.O. Box 340308
Hartford, CT 06134-0308
(860) 509-7588
Temporary Permit: 90 days from completion of nursing program. Temporary permit also available for endorsement applicants, valid for 120 days, nonrenewable; must hold valid license in another state. Fee is included in application fee.
State Board Fee: $90 R.N., $75 L.P.N.
Additional State Endorsement: $90 R.N., $75 L.P.N.
NCLEX Test Fee: $88
Re-Examination Limitations: May test no more than once every 91 days and no more than four times in one year
License Renewal: Every year, last day of birth month. $50 R.N., $30 L.P.N.
CEU Requirements: None

Delaware

Board of Nursing
Cannon Building, Suite 203
P.O. Box 1401
Dover, DE 19903
(302) 739-4522
Temporary Permit: 90 days from date of graduation pending results of first exam; endorsement applicants must hold valid license in another state. Fee is included in licensure fee.
State Board Fee: $84, $10 re-examination
Additional State Endorsement: $84
NCLEX Test Fee: $88
Re-Examination Limitations: Maximum four times per year for up to five years
License Renewal: February 28, May 31, and September 30. Every odd year R.N., every even year L.P.N.. $74
CEU Requirements: Nurses not actively employed in past five years must provide evidence of satisfactory completion of refresher program within the past 2 years, must have 1,000 hours employment in past five years or 400 hours in the past two years to renew; 30 contact hours every two years for R.N.; 24 contact hours for L.P.N.

District of Columbia

Nurses Examining Board
614 H Street NW, Room 904
Washington, DC 20001
(202) 727-7468
Temporary Permit: None
State Board Fee: $50
Additional State Endorsement: $40
NCLEX Test Fee: $88
Re-Examination Limitations: None
License Renewal: Every two years,
$48
CEU Requirements: Applicants for
reinstatement of a license must sub-
mit 12 contact hours for each year
after 6/30/90 that the applicant was
not licensed, up to maximum of 24
contact hours

Florida

Board of Nursing
4080 Woodcock Drive, Suite 202
Jacksonville, FL 32207
(904) 858-6940
Temporary Permit: 90 days pending
results of first exam; 120 days if by
endorsement. Fee is included in
licensure fee.
State Board Fee: $160 first time
Additional State Endorsement:
$175
NCLEX Test Fee: Included in state
board fee

Re-Examination Limitations:
None
License Renewal: Every two years,
odd year. $65
CEU Requirements: 25 contact
hours every two years. One credit
per month. Proof of training in HIV
and domestic violence by a provider
approved by the state of Florida.

Georgia

Board of Nursing
166 Pryor Street SW, Suite 400
Atlanta, GA 30303
(404) 656-3943
Temporary Permit: Six months if
by endorsement. Fee is included in
application fee.
State Board Fee: $40
Additional State Endorsement: $60
NCLEX Test Fee: $88 plus $9.25
when registering by telephone
Re-Examination Limitations: Three
years
License Renewal: January 31, every
even year. $40 if paid before
November 30, $60 after November 30.
CEU Requirements: None

Hawaii

Board of Nursing
P.O. Box 3469
Honolulu, HI 96801
(808) 586-3000
Temporary Permit: Pending results of first exam or completion of endorsement; may be repealed in one year. No fee
State Board Fee: $20
Additional State Endorsement: $70 or $115, depending on the year license is issued. Noted on application information sheet.
NCLEX Test Fee: $88
Re-Examination Limitations: Every 91 days.
License Renewal: June 30, every odd year. $90
CEU Requirements: None.

Idaho

Board of Nursing
280 North 8th Street, Suite 210
P.O. Box 83720
Boise, ID 83720-0061
(208) 334-3110
Temporary Permit: 90 days if by endorsement, $15
State Board Fee: $75
Additional State Endorsement: $75
NCLEX Test Fee: $88
Re-Examination Limitations: None

License Renewal: August 31, every two odd years. $45
CEU Requirements: None

Illinois

Dept. of Professional Regulation
320 W. Washington Street, 3rd fl.
Springfield, IL 62786
(217) 785-0800
Temporary Permit: Three-month approval letter
State Board Fee: $50
Additional State Endorsement: $50
NCLEX Test Fee: $88
Re-Examination Limitations: Three years from first writing to board
License Renewal: May 31 of every even year, R.N.; January 31 of every odd year, L.P.N.. $40
CEU Requirements: None

Indiana

State Board of Nursing
Health Professions Bureau
402 W. Washington Street, Room 041
Indianapolis, IN 46204
(317) 232-2960
Temporary Permit: 60 days if by endorsement, $10
State Board Fee: $30 R.N., $20 L.P.N..
Additional State Endorsement: $30 in, $10 out

NCLEX Test Fee: $88
Re-Examination Limitations: No limit; may retest every 91 days.
License Renewal: October 31, every odd year. $20
CEU Requirements: None

Iowa

Board of Nursing
1223 East Court
Des Moines, IA 50319
(515) 281-3255
Temporary Permit: 30 days if by endorsement. Fee is included in application fee.
State Board Fee: $60 R.N., $55 L.P.N.
Additional State Endorsement: $78
NCLEX Test Fee: $88
Re-Examination Limitations: None
License Renewal: Triennial, birth month. $63
CEU Requirements: 4.5 contact hours or 4.5 CEUs every three years

Kansas

State Board of Nursing
Landon State Office Bldg.
900 SW Jackson, Suite 551 S.
Topeka, KS 66612-1230
(785) 296-4929
Temporary Permit: Pending results of first exam, or no longer than 90 days from graduation; 120 days if by endorsement. Fee is included in application fee.
State Board Fee: $70 R.N., $45 L.P.N.
Additional State Endorsement: $70 R.N., $45 L.P.N.
NCLEX Test Fee: $88
Re-Examination Limitations: Unlimited number of times; after two years the applicant must provide an approved study plan.
License Renewal: Month of birth, every two years. $50
CEU Requirements: 30 contact hours every two years

Kentucky

Board of Nursing
312 Whittington Parkway, Suite 300
Louisville, KY 40222-5172
(502) 329-7000
Temporary Permit: No temporary permits are issued to new graduates. Six months if by endorsement. Fee is included in application fee.
State Board Fee: $80
Additional State Endorsement: $80
NCLEX Test Fee: $88
Re-Examination Limitations: None
License Renewal: October 31. Every even year R.N., every odd year L.P.N.. $65 active, $45 inactive

CEU Requirements: 30 contact hours every two years; two hours of the 30 hours must be AIDS CE-approved by the Kentucky Cabinet for Health Services. A one-time domestic violence requirement must be completed within three years of the date of initial licensing.

Louisiana

Board of Nursing
3510 North Causeway Boulevard, Suite 501
Metairie, LA 70002
(504) 838-5332
Temporary Permit: Pending results of first exam; 90 days if by endorsement. Fee is included in application fee.
State Board Fee: $35
Additional State Endorsement: $50 in, $15 out
NCLEX Test Fee: $88
Re-Examination Limitations: Four times in four years.
License Renewal: January 31, every year. $25
CEU Requirements: For all R.N.s; 5, 10, or 15 contact hours every year, based on employment

Maine

Board of Nursing
State House Station 158
Augusta, ME 04333
(207) 287-1133
Temporary Permit: 90 days. Fee is included in application fee.
State Board Fee: $60 R.N., $50 L.P.N.
Additional State Endorsement: $60 R.N., $50 L.P.N.
NCLEX Test Fee: $88
Re-Examination Limitations: None
License Renewal: Birthday, every two years. $40
CEU Requirements: None

Maryland

Board of Nursing
4140 Patterson Avenue
Baltimore, MD 21215
(410) 585-1900
Temporary Permit: 90 days, not renewable; no graduate nurse status, $25
State Board Fee: $50
Additional State Endorsement: $75
NCLEX Test Fee: $88
Re-Examination Limitations: None
License Renewal: Month of birth by the 28th day of each month, every year. $30
CEU Requirements: None

Massachusetts

Attn: Board of Registration in
Nursing
100 Cambridge Street
Boston, MA 02208
(617) 727-3074
Temporary Permit: No graduate
nurse status. No fee
State Board Fee: $166
Additional State Endorsement: $75
NCLEX Test Fee: Included in state
board fee.
Re-Examination Limitations: None
License Renewal: Birthday. Every
even year R.N., every odd year
L.P.N.; five-day grace period, $25
late fee. $40. Expanded role nurses,
$60.
CEU Requirements: 15 contact
hours every two years

Michigan

Board of Nursing
P.O. Box 30193
Lansing, MI 48909
(517) 335-0918
Temporary Permit: No longer avail-
able.
State Board Fee: $40
Additional State Endorsement: $40
NCLEX Test Fee: $88
Re-Examination Limitations: Six
attempts within three years

License Renewal: March 31, every
two years.
CEU Requirements: 25 credits every
two years

Minnesota

Board of Nursing
2829 University Avenue, SE #500
Minneapolis, MN 55414
(612) 617-2270
Temporary Permit: 60 days; one
year if by endorsement, $50
State Board Fee: $80
Additional State Endorsement: $80
NCLEX Test Fee: $88
Re-Examination Limitations: Once
every three months, for a maximum
of 4 times per year.
License Renewal: Birth month,
Every two years. $55
CEU Requirements: R.N.s, 24 con-
tact hours; L.P.N.s, 12 contact
hours every two years; R.N.s, 2-
hour course in infection control;
L.P.N.s, one-hour course on infec-
tion control.

Mississippi

Board of Nursing
1935 Lakeland Drive
Jackson, MS 39216-5014
(601) 987-4188
Temporary Permit: 90 days by endorsement, $25
State Board Fee: $60
Additional State Endorsement: $60
NCLEX Test Fee: $88
Re-Examination Limitations: None
License Renewal: December 31. Every even year R.N., every odd year L.P.N.. $50
CEU Requirements: NPs, 40 hours every two years; none for R.N.s and L.P.N.s.

Missouri

Board of Nursing
P.O. Box 656
Jefferson City, MO 65102
(573) 751-0681
Temporary Permit: Six months. Fee is included in application fee.
State Board Fee: $20 R.N., $11 L.P.N.
Additional State Endorsement: $30 R.N., $26 L.P.N.
NCLEX Test Fee: $88
Re-Examination Limitations: None
License Renewal: April 30, every two years R.N.; May 31, every two

years L.P.N.. $23 R.N., $19 L.P.N.
CEU Requirements: None

Montana

Board of Nursing
Arcade Building
111 North Jackson
P.O. Box 200513
Helena, MT 59620-0513
(406) 444-2071
Temporary Permit: 90 days. Fee is included in application fee.
State Board Fee: $70
Additional State Endorsement: $70
NCLEX Test Fee: $88
Re-Examination Limitations: None
License Renewal: December 31, every year. $40
CEU Requirements: None

Nevada

Board of Nursing
P.O. Box 46886
Las Vegas, NV 89114
(702) 688-2620
Temporary Permit: Four months, not renewable in 12-month period. Fee is included in application fee; $50 if not seeking permanent license
State Board Fee: $105 R.N., $95 L.P.N.
Additional State Endorsement: $105 R.N., $95 L.P.N.

NCLEX Test Fee: $88
Re-Examination Limitations: Three times, then only with remediation
License Renewal: Birthday, every two years (licensed as of 1/1/86). $100
CEU Requirements: All licensed nurses: 30 contact hours every two years at renewal

New Hampshire

Board of Nursing
Division of Public Health Services
P.O. Box 3898
Concord, NH 03302
(603) 271-2323
Temporary Permit: Six months or until results of first exam are received and license is issued, $20
State Board Fee: $80
Additional State Endorsement: $70
NCLEX Test Fee: $88
Re-Examination Limitations: None
License Renewal: Birthday, every two years. $60
CEU Requirements: Active in practice; 900 hours using nursing knowledge, judgment, and skills within four years immediately prior to application for renewal, endorsement, and reinstatement; 30 contact hours every to years at renewal.

New Jersey

Board of Nursing
P.O. Box 45010
Newark, NJ 07101
(973) 504-6430
Temporary Permit: Pending results of first exam; if working, must take within 45 days of graduation. No fee
State Board Fee: $50
Additional State Endorsement: $60
NCLEX Test Fee: $88
Re-Examination Limitations: Three times, only with remediation
License Renewal: December 31, every two years. $50
CEU Requirements: Advanced practice 30 contact hours every two years

New Mexico

Board of Nursing
4206 Louisiana NE, Ste. A
Albuquerque, NM 87109
(505) 841-8340
Temporary Permit: 24 weeks from graduation if application process is completed within 12 weeks of graduation; six months if by endorsement. Fee is included in application fee; must have NM employment verified.
State Board Fee: $90
Additional State Endorsement: $90
NCLEX Test Fee: $88

Re-Examination Limitations: None
License Renewal: Every two years from date of issue. $60
CEU Requirements: 30 contact hours every two years; NPs, 50 contact hours including 15 hours minimum in pharmacology every two years

New York

Board of Nursing State Ed. Dept.
Cultural Education Center
Albany, NY 12230
(518) 474-3843
Temporary Permit: Ten days after exam scores are posted, or up to one year, $35
State Board Fee: $120 (includes first license and 3-year registration) for R.N. and L.P.N., $112 per specialty area for NP
Additional State Endorsement: $120
NCLEX Test Fee: $88
Re-Examination Limitations: None
License Renewal: Triennial (licensed as of 9/1/83). $50
CEU Requirements: One-time requirement for registration; 2-hour course on child abuse; 4-hour course in infection control every four years

North Carolina

Board of Nursing
P.O. Box 2129
Raleigh, NC 27602
(919) 782-3211
Temporary Permit: Six months, not renewable. Fee is included in application fee.
State Board Fee: $50
Additional State Endorsement: $90
NCLEX Test Fee: $88
Re-Examination Limitations: No limit
License Renewal: December 31, every two years. $60
CEU Requirements: None

North Dakota

Board of Nursing
919 S. 7th Street, Suite 504
Bismarck, ND 58504
(701) 328-2000
Temporary Permit: 60 days pending results of first exam; 90 days if by endorsement. Fee is included in application fee.
State Board Fee: $75
Additional State Endorsement: $75
NCLEX Test Fee: $88
Re-Examination Limitations: Five attempts in five years
License Renewal: Every two years. $60 R.N., $50 L.P.N.

CEU Requirements: Nursing practice for relicensure must meet or exceed 500 hours within preceding five years.

Ohio

Board of Nursing
77 South High Street, 17th floor
Columbus, OH 43266-0316
(614) 466-3947
Temporary Permit: Endorsement—4 months. Fee is included in endorsement application fee.
State Board Fee: $50
Additional State Endorsement: $50
NCLEX Test Fee: $88
Re-Examination Limitations: Must wait three months
License Renewal: September 1, every odd year. $35
CEU Requirements: 24 hours for R.N. and L.P.N. in a 2-year period

Oklahoma

Board of Nursing
2915 Classen Boulevard, Suite 524
Oklahoma City, OK 73106
(405) 962-1800
Temporary Permit: 90 days, only for nurses seeking endorsement. Fee is included in application fee.
State Board Fee: $55
Additional State Endorsement: $55

NCLEX Test Fee: $88
Re-Examination Limitations: None
License Renewal: R.N. every even year by end of birth month. L.P.N. every odd year by end of birth month.
CEU Requirements: APN has prescriptive authority

Oregon

Board of Nursing, Suite 465
800 NE Oregon Street
Portland, OR 97232
(503) 731-4745
Temporary Permit: None
State Board Fee: $70
Additional State Endorsement: $50
NCLEX Test Fee: $88
Re-Examination Limitations: None
License Renewal: Birthday, every two years. $54 R.N., $55 NP. Prescriptive authority, $154 (must be renewed at same time). Late fees: $10 R.N. and NP.
CEU Requirements: 960 hours of practice within past five years

Pennsylvania

Board of Nursing
P.O. Box 2649
Harrisburg, PA 17105-2649
(717) 783-7142
Temporary Permit: 1 year maxi-

mum; examination results preempt permit, $20
State Board Fee: $35
Additional State Endorsement: $25
NCLEX Test Fee: $88
Re-Examination Limitations: None
License Renewal: Renewal date by license number every two years. $21 R.N., $16 L.P.N.
CEU Requirements: None

Rhode Island

Board of Nurse Registration and Nursing Education
Three Capitol Hill, Room 104
Providence, RI 02908
(401) 222-2827
Temporary Permit: Pending results of first exam but no longer than 90 days after graduation; 90 days if by endorsement. No fee.
State Board Fee: $75
Additional State Endorsement: $75 R.N., $50 L.P.N.
NCLEX Test Fee: $88
Re-Examination Limitations: None
License Renewal: March 1, every two years by license number
CEU Requirements: None

South Carolina

Board of Nursing
P.O. Box 12367
Columbia, SC 29210
(803) 896-4550
Temporary Permit: Pending results of first exam; 90 days if by endorsement, $10
State Board Fee: $65 R.N., $45 L.P.N.
Additional State Endorsement: $75
NCLEX Test Fee: $88
Re-Examination Limitations: Up to four times in 1 year, then must remediate
License Renewal: October 1–January 1, every year. $25
CEU Requirements: Minimum practice requirement 960 hours in preceding years

South Dakota

Board of Nursing
4300 S. Louise Ave., Suite C1
Sioux Falls, SD 57106-3124
(605) 362-2760
Temporary Permit: Pending results of first exam; 90 days if by endorsement, $15
State Board Fee: $60 R.N., $35 L.P.N.
Additional State Endorsement: $75 R.N., $50 L.P.N.

NCLEX Test Fee: $88
Re-Examination Limitations:
Maximum of four times per year, in three years postgraduation, then must requalify
License Renewal: Birthday, every two years. $55 (includes $10 for nurse education assistance loan fund)
CEU Requirements: Continuing practice requirement 140 hours/year or 480 hours/6 years

Tennessee

Board of Nursing
425 Fifth Avenue North
Cordell Hull Bldg., First Floor
Nashville, TN 37247-1010
(615) 532-5166
Temporary Permit: Six months if by endorsement, $10
State Board Fee: $85 R.N., $60 L.P.N.
Additional State Endorsement: $85
NCLEX Test Fee: $88
Re-Examination Limitations: Three years, then only with remediation.
License Renewal: Birthday, every two years. $50 R.N., $45 L.P.N.
CEU Requirements: Continued practice requirement over a five-year period.

Texas

Board of Nurse Examiners
P.O. Box 430
Austin, TX 78767
(512) 305-7400
Temporary Permit: 12 weeks to allow nurse to satisfy requirement, $15
State Board Fee: $50
Additional State Endorsement: $75 (includes temporary license)
NCLEX Test Fee: $88
Re-Examination Limitations: Three attempts within four years
License Renewal: Birthday, every two years. $35 (includes $5 for peer assistance)
CEU Requirements: 20 contact hours for two years

Utah

Board of Nursing
Div. of Professional Licensing
160 E. 300 South
Salt Lake City, UT 84114-6741
(801) 530-6628
Temporary Permit: None
State Board Fee: None
Additional State Endorsement: $50
NCLEX Test Fee: $88
Re-Examination Limitations:
Those who fail to pass exam within two years after completing educa-

tional program must submit plan of action for approval before retaking.
License Renewal: January 31, every odd year. $40
CEU Requirements: Must have practiced not less than 400 hours during two years preceding application for renewal; or have completed 30 contact hours or have practiced not less than 200 hours and completed 15 contact hours during two years preceding application for renewal

Vermont

Board of Nursing
109 State Street
Montpelier, VT 05609-1106
(802) 828-2396
Temporary Permit: Pending receipt of examination results or 90 days, whichever comes first. No fee
State Board Fee: $90
Additional State Endorsement: $60
NCLEX Test Fee: $88
Re-Examination Limitations: Board of nursing approval is needed after two times
License Renewal: Every odd year for R.N. (licensed as of 3/31/95 and L.P.N. (licensed as of 1/3/96). $60
CEU Requirements: None

Virginia

Board of Nursing
6606 West Broad Street, 4th floor
Richmond, VA 23230-12717
(804) 662-9909
Temporary Permit: None.
State Board Fee: $25
Additional State Endorsement: $50
NCLEX Test Fee: $88
Re-Examination Limitations: None
License Renewal: Birthday, every two years. $40
CEU Requirements: None

Washington

Nursing Commission
P.O. Box 1099
Olympia, WA 98507-1099
(360) 236-4702
Temporary Permit: None
State Board Fee: $65
Additional State Endorsement: $40 R.N., $69 L.P.N.
NCLEX Test Fee: $88
Re-Examination Limitations: Four times in two years; then must requalify
License Renewal: Birthday, every two years. $50.

CEU Requirements: Advanced registered nurse practitioner: 30 contact hours every two years with prescriptive authorization. 15 added hours in pharmacology as of 1/1/87

West Virginia

Board of Examiners for R.N.'s
101 Dee Drive
Charleston, WV 25311-1620
(304) 558-3596
Temporary Permit: Pending results of first exam but no longer than 90 days from graduation, new gradutates only; 90 days if by endorsement, $10
State Board Fee: $51.50
Additional State Endorsement: $30
NCLEX Test Fee: $88
Re-Examination Limitations:
Additional requirements are needed after two times
License Renewal: December 31, every year. $25
CEU Requirements:
Implementation in 1997. Thirty contact hours for first three years through 12/99; then 30 contact hours every two years

Wisconsin

Board of Nursing
P.O. Box 8935
Madison, WI 53708-8935
(608) 266-0145
Temporary Permit: Three months upon proof of graduation; three months if by endorsement; must take exam, $10.
State Board Fee: $47
Additional State Endorsement: $46 R.N., $48 L.P.N.
NCLEX Test Fee: $88
Re-Examination Limitations: 91-day wait
License Renewal: February 28, every even year. $46 R.N., $40 L.P.N.. $25 late fee
CEU Requirements: None

Wyoming

Board of Nursing
2020 Carey Avenue, Suite 110
Cheyenne, WY 82002
(307) 777-7601
Temporary Permit: 90 days from date of issue. Fee is included in application fee.
State Board Fee: $100, plus $60 fingerprint fee.
Additional State Endorsement: $115 R.N., $105 L.P.N. plus $60 fingerprint fee

NCLEX Test Fee: $88
Re-Examination Limitations: Retest maximum 10 times within 5 years of graduation. 90-day wait between tests.
License Renewal: Month of birth, every even year. $80 R.N., $70 L.P.N.
CEU Requirements: 500 hours in past 2 years, 1600 hours in the past 5 years. If not, 20 hours of contact for the past 2 years

Appendix C

A Special Note for International Nurses

If you are not from the United States but are interested in learning more about American nursing, wish to practice in the United States, or are exploring the possibilities of attending an American nursing school for graduate study, Kaplan can help you.

To function as a registered nurse in the United States, it is necessary for you to become licensed as a R.N. by a state board of nursing. Many U.S. state boards of nursing require internationally-educated nurses to obtain a certificate from the Commission on Graduates of Foreign Nursing Schools (CGFNS) before applying for initial licensure as a registered nurse. The process of obtaining a CGFNS certificate includes (1) a comparison of your nursing education credentials to what is required of US nursing graduates, (2) passing the CGFNS exam that tests nursing knowledge, and (3) obtaining a score of 540 on the TOEFL (Test of English as a Foreign Language). Kaplan offers comprehensive courses of study to help you pass the CGFNS and TOEFL exams. To obtain course information please call 1-800-KAP-TEST. Outside the U.S.A. please call 1-212-262-4980.

Applications for the CGFNS exam are free and can be obtained by calling CGFNS at (215) 349-8767. To find out about a particular state's requirements for international nurses, call that state's board of nursing and request an application packet for initial licensure as an internationally educated nurse. The phone numbers and addresses for each of the State Boards of nursing in the United States are listed in Appendix B of this book.

Once you as have a CGFNS certificate, it is necessary for you to take and pass the NCLEX exam (National Council Licensure Examination). You should apply to the state board of nursing where you wish to practice nursing to take the NCLEX exam. Kaplan has a comprehensive course and review products to help you pass this exam. To obtain course information, please call 1-800-KAP-TEST. Outside the U.S.A. please call 1-212-262-4980.

Additional Resources for International Students and Professionals

In addition to nursing courses, Kaplan provides international students and professionals programs to develop the English language skills necessary to study or work in the U.S.A. Course offerings include intensive English, Pre-MBA studies and standardized exam preparation for such exams as the SAT, TOEFL, GMAT, and GRE. With campus and city centers across the U.S.A., Kaplan has a location perfect for everyone. Call 1-800-527-8378. Or, outside the U.S.A., call 1-212-262-4980.

Kaplan is authorized under U.S. federal law to enroll nonimmigrant alien students.

Notes

Notes

Notes

Notes

Notes

Notes

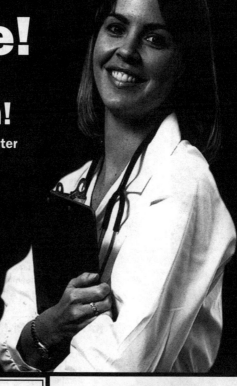
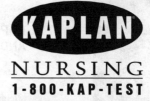

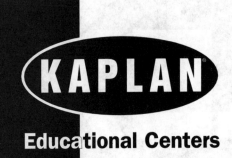

Educational Centers

Kaplan Educational Centers is one of the nation's premier education companies, providing individuals with a full range of resources to achieve their educational and career goals. Kaplan, celebrating its 60th anniversary, is a wholly owned subsidiary of the Washington Post Company.

TEST PREPARATION AND ADMISSIONS CONSULTING

Kaplan's nationally recognized test prep courses cover more than 20 standardized tests, including secondary school, college, and graduate school entrance exams and foreign language and professional licensing exams. In addition, Kaplan offers private tutoring and comprehensive one-to-one admissions and application advice for students applying to law and business school.

SCORE! EDUCATIONAL CENTERS

SCORE! after-school learning centers help K-8 students build confidence, academic and goal-setting skills in a motivating, sports-oriented environment. Our cutting-edge interactive curriculum continually assesses and adapts to each child's academic needs and learning style. Enthusiastic Academic Coaches serve as positive role models creating a high-energy atmosphere where learning is exciting and fun.

KAPLAN LEARNING SERVICES

Kaplan Learning Services provides customized assessment, education, and training programs to elementary and high schools, universities and businesses to help students and employees reach their academic and career goals.

KAPLAN PROGRAMS FOR INTERNATIONAL STUDENTS AND PROFESSIONALS

Kaplan services international students and professionals in the U.S. through *Access America*, a series of intensive English language programs. These programs are offered at Kaplan City Centers and four new campus-based centers in California, Washington and New York via Kaplan/LCP International Institute. Kaplan and Kaplan/LCP offer specialized services to sponsors including placement at top American universities, fellowship management, academic monitoring and reporting, and financial administration.

KAPLAN PUBLISHING

Kaplan Books, a joint imprint with Simon & Schuster, publishes titles in test preparation, admissions, education, career development and life skills; Kaplan and *Newsweek* jointly publish the popular guides, **How to Get Into College** and **How to Choose a Career & Graduate School**. *SCORE!* and *Newsweek* have teamed up to publish **How to Help Your Child Succeed in School**.

KAPLOAN

Students may obtain information and advice about educational loans for college and graduate school through **KapLoan** (Kaplan Student Loan Information Program). Through an affiliation with one of the nation's largest student loan providers, **KapLoan** helps direct students and their families through the often bewildering financial aid process.

KAPLAN INTERACTIVE

Kaplan InterActive delivers award-winning educational products and services including Kaplan's best-selling **Higher Score** test-prep software and sites on the internet (http://www.kaplan.com) and America Online. Kaplan and Cendant Software jointly offer educational software for the K-12 retail and school markets.

KAPLAN CAREER SERVICES

Kaplan helps students and graduates find jobs through Kaplan Career Services, the leading provider of career fairs in North America. The division includes **Crimson & Brown Associates**, the nation's leading diversity recruitment and publishing firm, and **The Lendman Group and Career Expo,** both of which help clients identify highly sought-after technical personnel, and sales and marketing professionals.

COMMUNITY OUTREACH

Kaplan provides educational resources to thousands of financially disadvantaged students annually working closely with educational institutions, not-for-profit groups, government agencies and other grass roots organizations on a variety of national and local support programs. Kaplan enriches local communities by employing high school, college, and graduate students, creating valuable work experiences for vast numbers of young people each year.

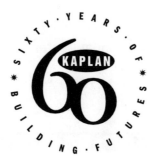

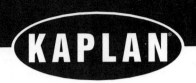

Want more information about our services, products, or the nearest Kaplan center?

1 **Call our nationwide toll-free numbers:**

1-800-KAP-TEST for information on our live courses, private tutoring and admissions consulting
1-800-KAP-ITEM for information on our products
1-888-KAP-LOAN* for information on student loans

(outside the U.S.A., call **1-212-262-4980**)

2 **Connect with us in cyberspace:**

On AOL, keyword:"Kaplan"
On the World Wide Web, go to: **http://www.kaplan.com**
Via e-mail: info@kaplan.com

3 **Write to:**

Kaplan Educational Centers
888 Seventh Avenue
New York, NY 10106